Pengui
Positiv

Susan Quilliam was born i............ .... read Psychology and English at Liverpool University. After a period of teaching she moved to London where she now works as a freelance writer. A trainer and counsellor, she has many years of experience working with women and those under stress. She has written eleven study guides in the Penguin Passnotes series, and is the author, with Ian Grove-Stephensen, of *Love Strategies* (1987), and *How to Stay in Love* (1988), practical guides to successful relationships.

SUSAN QUILLIAM

POSITIVE SMEAR

PENGUIN BOOKS

PENGUIN BOOKS

Published by the Penguin Group
27 Wrights Lane, London W 8 5 T Z, England
Viking Penguin Inc., 40 West 23rd Street, New York, New York 10010, U S A
Penguin Books Australia Ltd, Ringwood, Victoria, Australia
Penguin Books Canada Ltd, 2801 John Street, Markham, Ontario, Canada L 3 R 1 B 4
Penguin Books (N Z) Ltd, 182–190 Wairau Road, Auckland 10, New Zealand

Penguin Books Ltd, Registered Offices: Harmondsworth, Middlesex, England

First published by Penguin Books 1989
1 3 5 7 9 10 8 6 4 2

Copyright © Susan Quilliam, 1989
Photographs by Maggie Murray
Illustrations by Audrey Besterman
All rights reserved

Made and printed in Great Britain by
Richard Clay Ltd, Bungay, Suffolk
Filmset in Linotron 202 Plantin by
Rowland Phototypesetting Ltd, Bury St Edmunds, Suffolk

CONTENTS

Part IV: The Resources

ACKNOWLEDGEMENTS

———————

In preparing the acknowledgement list for a book of this kind, in which many people have contributed time, energy and skill, there is always the fear that someone has been left out. So I would like to begin with a thank-you to everybody who helped, whether or not their name is mentioned!

I should like to thank all the women who were willing to share their experiences and emotions with me, both those named below and those who preferred not to be named, as well as their friends and families.

Alain Allard, Andrew Woolley, Catherine O'Neill, Cedric, Diana, Dorothy Newton, Elizabeth Butters, Emma Allard, Evelyn Marsden, Frances, Heather Robinson, Hilda, Ian, Jane, Jane Ginsborg, Janet Wild (RGN), Janice, Joanne Hailey, Judith Roche, Julia Tozer, Julie, Lily Hopkins, Pat Kirwan, Rachel Woolley, Sue Linge, Sue Robaczynski, Viki Mills.

My thanks to these people and organizations for giving me their specialist advice and support:

Abnormal Smear Care Group of the Long Eaton and District Volunteer Bureau, Penny Brohn, Bristol Cancer Help Centre; Eleanor Brown; Alice Burns and the Women's National Cancer Control Campaign; Alison Carmichael, Institute of Oncology, Marie Curie Cancer Care; Annabel Geddes, Women Against Cervical Cancer; The Gynaecological Nursing Forum of the Royal College of Nursing; Sally Haslett; Amanda Kelsey, CancerLink; Dr Ann McPherson; Anthony C. Silverstone, Consultant Gynaecologist, University College Hospital; Elizabeth Skinner, Cancer Research Campaign; Donald Stevens, New Approaches to Cancer; Yvonne Terry, BACUP; the Health Editors of *Time Out* and *City Limits*; Patrick Walker, Consultant Gynaecologist, The Royal Free Hospital; Dr Jan de Winter, Emeritus Senior Consultant in Radiotherapy and Oncology, Royal Sussex County Hospital Brighton, Founder Director of Clinic for Cancer Prevention Advice Brighton; The Women's Health and Reproductive Rights Information Centre; Glenis Burgess, Mary Cooper, Nancy McKeith of Yorkshire Women's Video; Dr Penny Ward for proofing the manuscript, Cynthia Alves for co-ordinating the administration, Pam Dix and Jenny Condie of Penguin Books for their superb support and editing, and Ian Grove-Stephensen for helping it to happen. A final acknowledgement to Mr Albert Singer and the staff of the Royal Northern Hospital for treating me when I had a positive smear diagnosed, and for their very particular contribution in motivating me to write this book.

INTRODUCTION

Thirty thousand women in England and Wales will have a positive smear this year. This book answers the questions they will ask.

Cancer of the cervix is an important disease, whose incidence could be reduced substantially, as it has been in the Scandinavian countries, if there were greater awareness of and commitment to the detection of early abnormalities. The cervical smear detects changes before cancer develops, at a time when simple treatment can restore the cervix to normal. Regular smears are therefore an essential element in preventative medicine for women.

The first section of the book deals with the initial reaction of the woman and her doctor to the diagnosis and discusses possible methods of treatment. The second part considers in detail the physiological processes involved in cervical malignancy. In the third section, women are shown how to develop a positive mental and physical attitude to the diagnosis and to their way of life. The fourth is a resources section.

The author realized the need for such a book when she herself had an abnormal cervical smear, and has extensively investigated the emotional and physical implications of the subject. This book is therefore of considerable interest to all women and to all individuals involved in female health care.

Carmel A. E. Coulter
Consultant in Radiotherapy and Oncology
St Mary's and the Middlesex hospitals

FIRST WORDS

When a woman has a positive smear, she faces issues
around her sexuality, her fertility and her mortality. (Dr.
P.W.)

On 19 December 1981, my world fell apart. Sitting on the steps of
my flat, I read and reread the slip of paper from my doctor that
informed me that I had a 'positive smear', and that I needed to
come and see him as a matter of urgency. I had no idea what this
meant. I knew that I had had a routine cervical smear a few weeks
ago, and had been expecting the result. I knew that both my
parents had died of cancer. And I also knew that my doctor, a
placid and reassuring man, had used the word 'urgent' in his letter.
I am, I think, an intelligent woman, possessed of a normal amount
of resourcefulness and ability. But faced with that small slip of
paper, I broke down and sobbed uncontrollably.

What happened to me then was fairly typical of what happens to
women after they have had a positive smear. I went 'urgently' to my
doctor, who referred me for further examination. I saw a consultant, who assured me that my condition was minor – and then wrote
to me a week or two later saying that he had been mistaken. I did
need treatment; I had an advanced form of pre-cancer.

My reactions were very mixed: I sometimes felt an inner convic-
tion that what they had found was not pre-cancer but cancer, and
that I was going to die. Often I found myself remembering that this
was an illness of the cervix; how would it affect my sex life? What
about having children? I felt particularly powerless when faced
with medical professionals, strangely vulnerable to them because
the condition I had was sexual in nature.

A month later, having gone in to hospital once and been sent home again because I had a cold, I received my treatment. They used diathermy, a cauterization method that involved a general anaesthetic and left me for a week afterwards both sore and tired, and with bouts of nausea caused by the post-operation antibiotics.

My check-up pronounced me cured. One morning, a few months after the operation, I woke to find that I was feeling suddenly and inexplicably well, in a way that I hadn't done for years. I have had normal, negative smears ever since.

But that was not the end of it. I was, even at the time, taken aback by the strength of my reaction to what all the facts told me was a fairly minor medical problem. I was sometimes frightened that I would die, embarrassed that I had an illness in a sexual area, angry that it had happened to me. I had to stop and take stock of where I was, think through my life, my relationships, whether I wanted children. I had, more than at any time in my past, to fight for what I needed, medically and emotionally.

When the time came to write a book about having a positive smear, I took my own experience as a starting point. I wanted to know if other women had felt the same as I did – sometimes coping well, but sometimes confused and negative about the whole process. Had they asked the same questions I had about whether they would live, bear children, regain their sexuality? What sort of things did women need; what had I needed, five years ago, to help me cope – and more than cope – with what was happening?

I took a deep breath and began asking questions, of doctors, nurses, friends, partners – but above all, of the women themselves. I did over fifty interviews and took even more written evidence. The answers I got amazed me; a positive smear was, as one woman put it, 'far more than a cut on your arm'. Not all women felt like this. Some had regarded it as a mere ripple in their lives. But many had been concerned about the whole experience, many had had to stop and think, not just about whether they were free for the next hospital appointment, but about much deeper issues. As I continued, talking not only to patients but also to medical professionals, it became clear that the positive smear 'process' as it exists in Britain today is capable of raising questions about many areas in a woman's life.

Having raised them, however, it then fails to give clear-cut answers. The smear test is one of the few tests that can detect cancer in its pre-cancerous stages, when a 100 per cent cure is still possible. What worries many women, however, is the underlying urgency to most approaches to the problem, for the condition, once identified, needs monitoring to avoid the threat of serious illness. To complicate matters further, the cause of cervical cancer or pre-cancer is still debatable. The question of whether it is linked to sexual behaviour is particularly fraught, and in our society a positive smear result can provoke a barrage of value judgements that rebound not only on women but also on their partners. In short, when you have a positive smear, you open a whole Pandora's box of issues.

It seems to me, from the women I have spoken to, that saying such things is not scaremongering: in the first place, a woman who has a positive smear is one of the lucky ones – she has been spotted, and now has an almost 100 per cent chance of complete recovery; secondly, the extraordinary medical advances of recent years mean that women can now survive cervical cancer and the day-to-day medical competence means they are often treated effectively and with respect. So I am not suggesting to women that they sit and worry about what their positive smear result means. For I do not need to suggest this – women are already worrying quite enough.

After a positive smear, a woman faces a whole mixture of medical and emotional challenges, and to admit this is a step forward. For although we deny it, we are caught in a spiral of reassurance and mixed messages which inhibit real action. Only if we accept the fact that we have a problem can we begin to do something about it.

So what should we do? When I spoke to women, the central question I put was this: what do we as women (and those around us) need, in order to make sense of what is happening to us as we go through the positive smear process? And the answer I received was 'information . . . clarity . . . a knowledge of what is going to happen to me . . . a way of coping with my husband . . . a way of coping with myself . . . someone to tell me it's all right to cry . . . someone to tell me what all the mixed messages mean . . .'

In response to these needs then, a large part of this book deals with the physical aspects of cervical conditions: the biology, the causes, the treatments. But an equally large part of it is about the emotional aspects: how does what is happening affect how you feel about yourself? How does it affect your relationships with other people? How can you take control of what is happening? How can you make decisions about your health and your treatment? What skills and strengths can you develop as you move through the process? And how can you use positively the fact that it may make you stop and question things?

In particular, I have tried to accept that having a positive smear raises lots of questions, and that often there are no easy answers, only further challenges. A woman may not know what has caused her condition – but she can begin to look at where she might be vulnerable. She may have to question her sex life – but she can do this from choice and not because she is being blamed or frightened. She may feel helpless in her dealings with medical professionals – but she may also begin to realize that she has the power to become involved in the process of her own health.

The book, then, is divided into four parts. The section on *Process* takes a step-by-step look at what happens from the moment a positive smear result is received. The *Facts* section gives more 'hard-core' information, both on the biological aspects of the possible conditions a positive smear can indicate, and on the range of possible causes. This section could be read alongside the one on *Process* to gain some understanding of the medical aspects of what is happening. In the section on *Feelings* I have concentrated on the four key issues that women have raised when talking to me, and devoted a chapter to each. The final chapter in this section contains verbatim reports of women's own experiences. At the end of the book is a full *Resource* section of reading matter, people, films and other sources of information and support.

If you have just had a positive smear, use this book where and when appropriate, to guide you through the process. You may not want or need to read every chapter, and may prefer to concentrate on those which are relevant to you at the moment. If you are supporting someone who has just had a positive smear, then read the whole book, to prepare you for what might happen.

If your positive smear has been diagnosed as pre-cancerous, you will find most of the experiences you are likely to have charted in this book, along with the experiences of other women. If your positive smear has been diagnosed as meaning you have cancer, you will perhaps see this book as dealing with only the tip of your particular iceberg. You may want to go on to explore other sources or support groups that address your situation in more detail – and many such organizations are listed in the resource section at the back of this book.

If you have had a positive smear and are now recovered, then read this book to help you assimilate more fully, in retrospect, what happened. And if you have not yet had a positive smear, then remember that in all likelihood someone you know, maybe you yourself, will have one in the not-too-distant future.

If you are a medical professional, please read this book to remind you of what you already know – that it may be a 'minor medical issue, rarely serious' to you, but that for some of us, its discovery means that the world falls apart and needs to be put back together. If you are a medical policy maker, let the book stand as a cry for *more please* – more funds, more staff, more understanding, more attention.

Please also note that I am not a medical professional, despite being qualified in the field of emotional care. So I have not attempted to write a medical work, although all the factual sections of this book are medically sound. My aim has been to gain an understanding of the positive smear experience in a wider context than the purely physical, and to provide a book that complements other, more medically orientated ones.

A final thought. I am taking a risk in this book. I was warned against being too positive, of expecting too much of women. 'Women who are worrying won't want to hear about the positives,' I was told. 'They won't be able to learn from it.' It is undoubtedly true that for some women, having a positive smear may be just a ripple in their lives. But for many women, having a positive smear is a chance to stop and take stock – and if it is this for you, then I am sure you can learn from what is happening to you.

I believe that, even when (perhaps particularly when) we are at our most vulnerable, we can see clearly enough to learn from what is happening to us. A positive smear can make us totally rethink our relationship with ourselves, our bodies, other people, and our futures, and we can learn from that. We can take the good even from something unpleasant. We can grow. We can make a difficult experience into a vital part of our lives and our development as humans. We can turn a medical term on its head, and truly make a 'positive smear' a 'positive experience'.

1

HEARING THE NEWS

> My doctor rang to say I had a positive smear. It was as if a
> friend had rung me up with the news . . . (Linda)

You have had a smear test. Maybe because your Family Planning
Clinic includes one in your check-up; maybe because you have had
some bleeding and your doctor wants to make sure it is nothing
serious; maybe because this is a regular part of your health care –
for whatever reasons, you have had a smear test. You may or may
not know exactly what it means, or what the results mean. You may
or may not be aware of the implications, but you have had the test.

That was two weeks, four weeks, maybe two months ago.
Perhaps you have put it to the back of your mind, or perhaps it has
been concerning you a bit. 'I was pretending,' as one woman said,
'that I'd forgotten about it'. As the time goes by, you convince
yourself that there is nothing wrong, and nothing to worry about.

Then comes the news. It might arrive in that 'little brown
envelope', which when opened reveals a letter from your clinic or
doctor. You might be one of the lucky women whose doctor phones
them immediately the news comes through, or who gives them the
news in person. You might not be so lucky. 'I got a message on my
flatmate's telephone answering machine,' said Julia. Whichever
way you hear the news, this is the beginning.

The news

What will the news say? Usually, it will be a straightforward
statement that you have had a positive or 'abnormal' smear. It will
remind you that you had a smear, and when, and also tell you to call

into the doctor's surgery for a chat. Occasionally, your doctor or clinic will already have made a further appointment for you at a local hospital, and an appointment time and date will be given in the letter or phone call.

These are the bare bones of the news, but there are other messages locked into it too. Whoever is contacting you will want you to take your positive smear seriously, and might therefore use words like 'urgent' or 'at once'. Doctors may use medical terms such as 'infection', 'pre-cancer' or 'dyskaryosis'. It is also difficult sometimes, particularly during a phone call or consultation, to reconcile the businesslike message with what seems to be bad news. You may wonder what is really happening.

Some of the best messages contain a personal note from the doctor to you. Evelyn's doctor 'rang me immediately and said, "Look my dear, it's important that you go and have this seen to." I really appreciated that.' Doctors often do realize that women need to know what is happening and try to provide some understanding and reassurance right away. One woman's doctor wrote: 'Remember that smear tests are there to pick up changes before they get serious.' (Julie).

Some doctors are simply less sensitive, but you need to realize right from the start that at the other end of this news is a doctor who is human too. If s/he hasn't taken the time to word the message kindly or carefully, then that is his/her problem. It doesn't have to be yours.

First reactions

Many women report feeling shock as their first reaction: 'I just rushed into my flatmate's room and shrieked at him.' (Janet). Other women cope at first, and panic later: 'I kept thinking it was nothing to worry about; then I woke up in the middle of the night and thought – this must mean I'm dying.' (Diana). So if you are worried, if you have heard that a positive smear can mean treatment or serious illness and are panicked by this, then you are not alone. Many other women feel the same way.

At this stage, you may be unsure of how to react. You may not know what having a positive smear is all about: 'It's so totally unknowable. You can't conceive of what it could actually mean.' (Rosemary). However you may be able to take the news calmly. If so, and if you can mobilize yourself into effective practical action, then this is the best possible way to be. Being calm, cool and powerfully active is going to get you furthest, fastest.

Other people

Other people around you when you receive the news will have to cope with you. If you do turn to them for support, remember two things. Firstly, if they don't know you well enough, they will find it difficult to give you exactly what you want. If a message reaches you at work, for example, other people might not know how to handle it. Illness, particularly sexual illness, stirs up strange things in people. It can also be appropriate to delay your reaction. I got my letter an hour before an important dinner party. After the first solitary weep, I decided not to tell my partner until after the party, when I could get the support I wanted for as long as I wanted. But also remember that other people are often only too glad to help. And other people may well learn from you that they too can ask for support when they need it.

What to do?

You have had the news, the first reactions are over, and you now need to begin to assimilate what is happening, and decide what to do next.

This is not something to be done with acquaintances or casual workmates. For this you will need a friend, your partner, your Mum. If none of these are available, and you need to talk, you can contact a counselling network that will give you support over the phone; the Resource section in this book has plenty of ideas.

What are the issues you need to think through? The basic fact is that you have had a positive smear. This can mean a number of things. It could mean that you have a minor infection of the vagina or of the cervix which can be treated easily. It is also possible that you have an early pre-cancerous condition of the cervix which may need simple treatment or no treatment at all. There is a very slight possibility that you might have cancer, and if so there is an even slighter possibility that this might mean radical surgery.

It is easy at this stage for you, or other people, to suspect that you do have cancer and that you are going to die. There can also be a temptation to convince yourself that the doctors have made a mistake and that you can ignore the whole thing. Both of these possibilities are very unlikely. The truth is that you probably don't have cancer. It is also true that very few positive smear results are incorrect.

Of course, you don't *have* to go to the doctor or the hospital. No one is going to chase after you if you rip up the letter, ignore the phone call and pretend it never happened. Quite a few of the women I talked to considered doing just that. But remember this. Someone, somewhere, has noticed that you are not as healthy as you could be. They have told you. They have given you the chance to do something about it. If they hadn't, your condition could be getting progressively worse and you would have no choice in the matter.

So maybe what you at first thought of as bad news is in fact good news.

2

WHAT NEXT?

_____

> My consultant looked at me and said, 'I think you may
> have a problem . . .' (Viki)

After you hear the news of your positive smear the next step can
vary enormously. Your doctor may have arranged an examination
for you at the local hospital. If so, turn to Chapter 3 where I
describe this procedure. It is more likely that your doctor will see
you first, in order to talk about your smear result.

The letter from your GP or Family Planning Clinic will probably
have included an appointment date and time. If not, you have a
choice; to go and see your doctor, or to ring and ask to speak to
her/him on the phone to discuss your case. It is likely that the
doctor will prefer to see you in person, so don't be disappointed or
worried if the receptionist asks you to make an appointment. It
doesn't mean that the news is bad – your doctor simply thinks that
seeing you in person will be more helpful.

Getting the results

Whether you see your doctor or speak on the phone, s/he is ideally
placed to give you information about your case. By this time,
particularly if you have been reading this book, you will probably
have a good basic knowledge of what a positive smear means. If
not, then ask your doctor to explain this to you.

If you haven't yet looked at the section of this book that
deals with the facts about cervical conditions, I suggest you do
so now, since you may find it useful for understanding what
follows.

Smear result

The doctor will probably begin by telling you what your smear
result is. The result will have been passed on to your doctor by
means of a standard form, giving details of any abnormal changes
in the cells and any other information picked up during the smear
test. Remember that the doctor won't be able to tell you at this
stage whether you have a serious condition, or give you any details
about the condition you have; the smear test doesn't reveal this.
However, depending on what degree of dyskaryosis you have, the
doctor will be able to advise you whether to have a further
examination. Very often, with mild dyskaryosis, you won't be
referred for an examination. Instead, the doctor will ask you to
come back in three or six months for a repeat smear. With
moderate or severe dyskaryosis, and sometimes with mild dyskaryosis, if you have other symptoms, or a family history of cervical
problems, the doctor will usually arrange a hospital appointment
for you. S/he may do that there and then over the phone.

The doctor will probably give you a letter to post or take to the
hospital. 'Doesn't everyone steam the envelope open?' asked one
woman – and you will have to decide whether you want to or not!
Remember that it is your right to know what the doctors think your
condition is, but also that there are better ways of finding out than
being faced with a technical letter you can misunderstand. If you do
want straight answers, try asking your doctor or consultant – at least
that way you will have the chance to ask questions and have them
answered, obtain information, and possibly even some support.

Often, this is all that a doctor does at this stage: gives you any
information you need, and refers you to a specialist. The visit to the
doctor might be very short indeed. Very occasionally, particularly
if you have complained of particular symptoms and this has been
the reason for your smear test, s/he will give you an internal
examination. You probably will have had one before, but if not
there's a fuller description of what it entails on page 23.

Infections

Sometimes, other cervical tests will have been done at the
same time as your smear test. If an infection or virus has been

found, your doctor may take this opportunity to tell you about it.

Possible infections are thrush (Candida) or trichomoniasis. You will probably be given cream to insert in your vagina, or tablets to take. If you have a virus, such as the wart or herpes virus, you may have to go to a special clinic to have it treated and your doctor will give you details of this. Other chapters of this book include sections on infections and viruses and how they are treated. If you do have an infection, it may have made the smear result unclear and your doctor will ask you to have a repeat smear when the infection has been treated successfully.

Asking questions

Your doctor will usually give you all the information I have mentioned. It is useful, however, to take with you a check-list of questions to ask in case the doctor misses something you want to know about. Women I spoke to asked this kind of question during their visit:

> *What is my smear test result?*
> *What severity of dyskaryosis have I got?*
> *Is there any other evidence to indicate what my condition is?*
> *Is there any sign of infection? A virus?*
> *Do I need to see a consultant? When? Where?*
> *How will the appointment be made?*
> *Do I need to come back to you for a repeat smear? When?*
> *Should I make the appointment now?*

Getting support

Whether you see your doctor in person or speak on the phone, you may feel concerned when you contact her/him. You may want to talk about your situation and be reassured. You have to face the fact that some doctors will be quite happy to give you the information you need, but feel uneasy if you ask for counselling or support. In an ideal world, of course, GPs would have the opportunity and the energy to spend time with you and let you express your worries.

Some of them do: 'My doctor was wonderful; he knew I'd been

depressed recently, and told me he accepted that I'd be worried and that this was a bad time for a positive smear to have happened.' (Julie).

If your doctor is like this, then do confide any fears you have in him/her; s/he knows your medical and personal history and is in an ideal situation to help you. If not, then the responsibility is with you again, and you will have to find any emotional support you need elsewhere.

Afterwards

Repeat smear

After your visit to the doctor, you may not need to attend a hospital, but will have been asked to return for a repeat smear after a short interval. It is just as important (probably more so) to go for this smear as to go for the first one. Just because you have had a test doesn't mean to say that you are now safe for another three years; if the original test results were unclear, you need to have another as soon as you can.

Even if your doctor or FPC have said they will contact you when your next smear is due, this is never enough. They may forget, their records may go missing, or lightning may strike! If it does, and you miss a repeat smear, they won't suffer. You will.

As you leave the surgery or clinic, jot down in a diary the date when your repeat smear is due and mark in a date a few days before to remind you to arrange it. The best time to go for a smear is at the mid-point of your menstrual cycle – that is, about twelve to sixteen days after the first day of your period. When the repeat smear is done, make sure you find out the result; leave a stamped addressed envelope or ask when the result is likely to be in and ring back then. In this situation, where one smear has shown the need for a regular check on your health, you have every reason to have another.

Waiting

After visiting the doctor, you will probably know that the next stage is your hospital appointment. Here is where you may begin to learn the true (double) meaning of the word 'patient'. Waiting lists for such appointments can vary – depending on what your condition is and what part of the country you are in – from a few days to several months. You might be lucky and get an appointment fairly soon; this doesn't necessarily mean that you have a serious illness. Remember that doctors make their decisions about when to see you by considering the severity of your smear and your past medical history. I was seen within three days owing to the fact that both my parents had died of cancer, and despite the fact that at the time I only had mild dyskaryosis. If you develop any unusual bleeding or badly-smelling discharge, you will probably be seen quickly.

On the other hand, you may know that you have months to wait before you are examined and diagnosed, and this is very hard indeed. You may wonder whether your condition is getting worse, particularly as you don't yet know for sure what is the matter with you. Everyone I spoke to mentioned how difficult it was simply to wait: 'You never know what will happen . . . and you imagine the worst.' But remember that up to 50 per cent of women who are referred for examination after one mildly abnormal smear will need no treatment at all – and that it is highly unlikely if you do need treatment that your condition will deteriorate badly while you wait.

Also remember that waiting is not a passive occupation. There are many things you can do to help yourself while you wait. One thing to do is to check that your appointment has been made. One woman I spoke to waited three months for her appointment, only to find that her GP's letter had been mislaid; her phone call alerted the hospital staff and she got an appointment soon after. There is no need to haunt the hospital, but it's worth asking your GP what the normal waiting time is and when he expects you to get an appointment. You can then ring the hospital when that time period has elapsed.

The other thing to do is to muster your forces. Get well-informed – read this book and any others in the Resource section that interest you. Spend time with people who can support you, as suggested in other chapters of this book. Build up your general health and well-being; whatever is the matter with you, you'll cope with the result far better if you are healthy and relaxed: 'I set up my own support system by doing intense relaxation, swimming, walking slowly . . . to strengthen my heart and relax me.' (Julie).

Finally, while you wait, keep your eyes and ears out for other women in the same situation. You'll be amazed at how many there are. One woman likened it to being pregnant: 'you find everyone else is too!' If you contact these other women, you can talk to them, support them and be supported by them.

As with pregnancy, the waiting is often the hardest part.

3

THE EXAMINATION

I got the works – the questions, the menstrual history,
even a breast examination. It was great! (Julie)

In the positive smear process, hospital appointments are a bit like
milestones; you seem to spend all your time waiting for, thinking
about and heading for the next one. After the positive smear news
itself, the next milestone will probably be a further examination.
During the examination, the doctor will look at the evidence of
your positive smear, and then do some further tests to find out
what, if anything, is wrong.

Further examination can be carried out in a number of ways and
which process you go through will depend very much on the area
you live in and the resources that are available there. In addition,
some methods of examination also include – or are used as methods
of – treatment.

The steps described below, as with all medical examinations and
treatments, may not be carried out in quite this order. Hospitals
differ one from another in the way they go about examining – each
has its own routine. So be prepared for things to happen differently
for you. What follows is a basic framework into which you can fit
your own experience. It also provides some guidelines about basic
things which might occur later on in your treatment. Preparation,
coping with waiting rooms, what happens in an internal examination – all these are constant throughout the process. Remember
what is said about them here for reference later on. After your wait,
this next step seems like the light at the end of a long tunnel, though
you might feel scared and apprehensive about it.

There are two things you could feel apprehensive about: what the examination will be like, and its results. You may even find that all your negative feelings are being loaded on to one of these things, so that if asked, you will claim to be scared stiff about the examination – but in fact it is the results that really worry you.

Types of examination

There are three main types of examination used to investigate further. You may have just one before treatment, or you may need more than one. Some Health Authorities don't have the facilities to do certain types of examination, so you may not have a choice.

Colposcopy and punch biopsy: these are normally done at the same appointment, often in Out-patients. In a colposcopy the doctor looks at your cervix through a microscope on a stand; a punch biopsy involves taking a small sample of cells from your cervix for later examination.

Fractional curettage and biopsy: after a biopsy, the surface of your cervix is scraped and samples of cells are taken for later examination. This is often followed by a cauterization treatment, as described in Chapter 6, to treat as well as examine you. Since this is carried out under general anaesthetic, it usually entails an overnight stay in hospital.

Cone biopsy: a cone of tissue is taken from the cervix, and this is often in itself enough to remove the abnormal cells, as well as diagnose them. However if the cone biopsy shows invasive cancer, you will need further treatment. This also usually involves a general anaesthetic and is used to investigate conditions where the abnormal cells have spread further.

Curettage and cone biopsy are both minor operations that entail a short stay in hospital, and are often also methods of treatment. Because of this, I have chosen to deal with them in more detail later in this book in the sections on treatment. So if in your Health Authority, it is normal to examine and investigate your condition through these methods, you may find it appropriate to turn to the relevant sections of the book now.

Which is the best sort of examination? Colposcopy is often seen as a better option, perhaps because it involves only an out-patient visit. There is no proof, however, that any one of these types of examination work better, and the curettage and cone biopsy can often include treatment as well – killing two birds with one stone. So there is no need to feel hard done by if your area doesn't have a colposcopy clinic.

Also remember that even after a colposcopy, if the abnormal cells are far up the cervical canal, you might need to have further examination by one of the other methods.

Preparations – at home

There are lots of ways that you can prepare for the examination. You may want to plan what to wear; a skirt is most sensible, since you can just slip off your underclothes when you are examined. Do check that your appointment doesn't clash with your period, for, as one woman I interviewed found to her cost, hospitals won't carry out some internal examinations if you are bleeding: 'I turned up, waited two hours, and then didn't even see a doctor when they heard I was having my period.'

You might like to have your partner or a friend with you at the hospital. Some things to consider when deciding who to take with you are the following: Who will help me to feel as good as I can before and after the examination? Who will allow me to be myself, and express my feelings if I want to? Who can stand up to the doctors and ask the questions I want asked, if I'm feeling groggy or intimidated?

Once you have found someone to go with you (and made sure they can go on the day of your appointment), you might like to spend some time with them, talking about how you feel and how you might want them to support you. Also spend some time making out a list of questions you want to ask the doctor. Throughout this chapter – and indeed throughout the book – I will be suggesting questions for you to ask, and you can add specific ones of your own.

Preparations – at the hospital

It is likely that your examination will be at a local hospital, in the Out-patients Gynaecological Clinic. It is possible, though unlikely unless you live in London or Glasgow, that your GP or Family Planning Clinic will be able to do the examination themselves.

When you arrive at the hospital and find your way to the clinic mentioned on your appointment card, you will probably have to check in at the reception desk after which you will probably have to wait. Many women I talked to complained about the waiting times for all kinds of diagnosis and treatment. This is certainly not something unique to gynaecological clinics – but waiting is always soul-destroying when you are waiting to hear what is wrong.

'All these women sitting round, too frightened to talk to one another', was how one interviewee described it. Perhaps there is a better way, if we realize that every woman there is probably in the same position as ourselves – or further down the treatment line. Talking to them can help you feel better, and make all of us feel less alone. A waiting-room full of women supporting each other by exchanging information, reassurance and help is a power-house of useful energy; tap into it if it exists, and if not, be the one to start it.

To undress or not

Once you are called by the nurse, you will have to negotiate the problem of undressing. Exactly what this involves will vary from hospital to hospital and from doctor to doctor. One doctor I saw insisted on seeing all his patients fully dressed before any examination because 'it creates an atmosphere of respect'. Not all hospitals are so enlightened, however: there are many horror stories of women clad in short white ward gowns 'with the back flapping open to show my bottom', having to wait on wooden seats for hours, embarrassed and chilly.

If you find yourself in this situation, you have two choices. You can refuse point blank to undress completely, and insist on being examined with just your briefs and tights off. If anyone argues, call in your friend or partner as support and simply stay calm and friendly – without removing your clothes. Or you can tell the nurse that you are very happy to undress, but will only do it just before the doctor is ready to see you. Ask her/him to let you know which patient is seeing the doctor before you, and then wait fully dressed until that patient goes in. Then get changed. The hour spent fully dressed and therefore feeling less vulnerable will be well worth it.

A final tip – whether you go in to see the doctor dressed or undressed, make sure you have your briefs with you, since you may need them later in order to wear a sanitary towel.

Meeting the consultant

Don't be overawed by any medical professional. Ask for your friend or partner to be there if you want them to be, and remember that it is worth your while to create an equal relationship right from the start. You can begin to do this by asking some questions right away. Some questions that women I talked to asked at this point were these:

> *What is your name? What sort of doctor are you? What job do you do in the hospital?*
> *What is the nurse's name? Will she stay in the room with me?*
> *What has my GP said to you in his letter?*
> *Are you going to do another smear? Colposcopy? A punch biopsy?*
> *Will there be anyone else in the room while I'm being examined?*

The last question can be more relevant than it seems: Julie's doctor began to examine her while students were in the room. She objected to this, and requested that they leave, which they did. You may feel, like Julie, that your medical condition and your body are something you only want to share with the doctor and nurse. On the other hand, you may like to let students learn from your situation. Whatever the case, you have a right to ask for what you want.

Doctor's questions

At this stage, the doctor will probably have some questions to ask you. They will often be about your gynaecological history to help the doctor understand what is going on in your cervix, and to have a context in which to interpret what s/he is seeing when s/he examines you. It is therefore worth answering them as fully as possible. You could perhaps prepare for them beforehand by making sure you know such things as: the date of your last period; the dates of your pregnancies; whether you are pregnant at the moment; whether there is any history of cancer in your family.

Some questions might embarrass you, however, and you may not want to answer them: the age at which you first had intercourse, or the number of sexual partners you have had are personal issues and you may think of them as things you want to keep to yourself. It is worth asking whether the doctor *needs* to know the answers to these questions in order to diagnose your condition. While it is very likely that s/he does, it is also possible that the questions are part of a larger issue – perhaps gathering information for a survey. Such surveys are of great use in detecting trends in cervical conditions and cancer, and it is important that women take part in them, but of course they are not related to your cure. So if a question causes you particular embarrassment, it is worth checking whether you really do need to reply to it.

Figure 1. A speculum is a metal instrument which looks like two shoe horns joined together.

The internal examination

The doctor will usually have read your notes and looked at the results of your positive smear. Then s/he will give you an internal examination. You will most likely have had one before, when you had your smear, but here is a detailed description. If you need further treatment, then you will have many more internals to come.

First you need to get into a position where the doctor can see inside your cervix. This usually means lying flat on your back on an examining couch with your legs raised and parted. There are special stirrups for your legs to rest on, which can be 'twigs on sticks' as one woman described them, or canvas or plastic slings into which your legs fit. This position can be off-putting; it may also make you feel vulnerable. But one woman's realization could help: 'Remembering that I was in charge helped a lot. I kept telling

Figure 2. As the speculum is eased apart, it opens your vagina so that the doctor can see inside it.

myself that I had chosen to be there because I wanted to be healthy – and that that meant I was in control.' (Tracey).

If you feel uncomfortable, do say so, and get the leg-rests adjusted. Feeling embarrassed does not mean you are what one interviewee called 'a nuisance patient'; lots of women feel this way, though do remember that to the doctor, you are an interesting cluster of cells, not a body s/he is emotionally or sexually aware of.

When you are settled, the doctor will place a metal instrument called a speculum into your vagina. You will almost certainly have had one used in your smear test. The speculum looks rather like two shoe horns joined together and as it is eased apart, it opens your vagina so that the doctor can see down to your cervix.

As with all these examinations and treatments, there is no promise that this will not be uncomfortable; however it is usually just cold. If you are uncomfortable, you might try asking your friend, or the nurse, to hold your hand or talk to you to distract you. One doctor in London has music playing and pictures on the ceiling of his colposcopy clinic – perhaps you should start a campaign for similar facilities in your area.

With your vagina open, the doctor will probably begin by taking another smear to see if the result is still the same. There have been cases of cervical conditions clearing up between one smear and the next.

The examination

Colposcopy

The next part of the examination is usually colposcopy. In colposcopy, the doctor looks at your cervix through a microscope on a stand. S/he examines the surface appearance of your cervix very closely, to see whether there are any signs of abnormality, and if there is any evidence of other problems. Remember that the doctor cannot tell from colposcopy how far or how deep the disease has spread, or whether it is cancerous.

First, s/he will put a liquid on your cervix: this may be a solution of acetic acid or iodine, so it could sting a bit. The abnormal areas turn a different colour, making them easier to see.

The doctor will then place the colposcope (microscope) at the entrance to your vagina, and will look closely at your cervix. In some clinics it is now possible for you to see what the doctor sees on closed circuit television; during my colposcopy, there was a blinding flash as they took photos: 'Smile, you're on *Candid Camera*!' was the comment.

Figure 3. A colposcope and an examining couch.

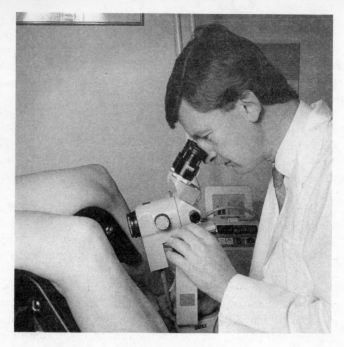

Figure 4. The doctor will look closely at your cervix.

The examination can take as long as ten or fifteen minutes, so don't panic if the doctor seems to be taking a close look. S/he will often tell you what s/he's doing as it happens. If not, and you want her/him to give you a running commentary, ask, though there will probably be a period when the doctor needs to concentrate and may not want to talk to you.

Punch biopsy

The next stage is usually for the doctor to take a small sample of the cervical cells for the laboratory to examine under a microscope. This is a normal thing to do, and does not mean you have cancer, so don't panic if the doctor talks about taking a 'biopsy'.

The doctor takes a tiny snippet of cells from your cervix, and will sometimes take more than one sample. It is hard to predict whether you will feel any pain at this stage, since it depends on a number of things: your doctor's sensitivity, your reaction to pain, the size of the sample. One woman described it as being: 'like a bad period pain', another said: 'it wasn't at all painful, and I'd been warned it would be.'

You might bleed however, and the nurse will probably give you a sanitary towel to put on afterwards. This is the reason for the earlier warning about making sure you have your briefs with you. Few things are more awkward than sitting clutching said towel while talking to the doctor, and at the same time 'feeling sticky underneath', as one woman put it.

When the biopsy is over, the doctor will usually go to wash her/his hands, while the nurse helps you out of the stirrups and down from the couch. If you haven't had your friend with you up to now, this is the time to ask him or her to come in while you talk to the doctor after the examination.

Often, at this point, the doctor has enough information to be able to tell you what is wrong. But sometimes, s/he may not be able to give you a definite diagnosis immediately after the examination. S/he may want to wait for the results of the biopsy or consult with another doctor. If you don't get a diagnosis at once, it certainly doesn't mean that something is seriously wrong. However, because examination and diagnosis are often two separate things, I have separated them into two chapters in this book.

Afterwards

Physical reactions

After the examination, your physical reactions might range from feeling nothing at all to feeling quite sore, especially after a biopsy. It is not a good idea to try to travel by bicycle, for obvious reasons, and it is probably wise to give yourself some time in case you need to sit down and collect yourself before you attempt the journey back home or to work.

On the other hand, you may be one of the lucky women who

simply bounces back and feels no after-effects. This is quite
normal; the important thing to remember is that if you do feel
physically vulnerable after the examination, this is quite normal,
too. If for any reason, after such an examination, you start bleeding
heavily when you are not due to have your period, then see your GP
or ring the hospital for advice.

A few women reported that after the examination, their consultant advised them not to have sex for a while. If your doctor says
nothing, then it is quite safe to have sex with your partner as soon as
you like. (In the context of this book, I use the words 'sex' or
'love-making' as doctors usually do, to mean penetration, which
can damage a vulnerable cervix. Do remember though, that enjoy-
able love-making need not involve penetration at all.)

Emotional reactions

Women's feelings about the examination also varied enormously:
'It didn't hurt, but it was bloody embarrassing,' said one woman.
'When you've had three children, it's not such an invasion of your
privacy,' said another.

If you dislike internal examinations, you may feel intruded
upon. If it was painful, you might feel angry or tearful. The
important thing to remember here is that simply because the doctor
is trying to help you doesn't mean that you have to feel totally
positive about everything.

You might, though, be one of the women I talked to who in fact
found something good in the experience. It helps if you can go into
the whole experience determined to find such things: were you
surprised at how supportive your friend was; satisfied with the
doctor's explanations; did you get on with the other women in the
waiting room?

Above all, did the doctor learn anything? Can s/he now, armed
with the information s/he has gained, go on to diagnose if anything
is wrong – and so begin to help you towards health?

4

THE DIAGNOSIS

> When they told me the diagnosis, I burst into tears. The doctor said 'Well, you must have known something was wrong.' (Sue)

The first thing to say about the diagnosis is that it won't necessarily take place at the same time as the examination. Often it does. The colposcopy over, the doctor can sit down with you and explain just what is happening, suggest treatment and send you away with all questions resolved. But it doesn't always happen like this.

The doctor may ask you to come back in a few weeks time. As always, the waiting list can vary, and I found examples of women delayed anything up to seven weeks for examination results. It is usual for women in this situation to be asked to come back to the same clinic, where they can see a consultant (though be warned, it might not be the same consultant); unlike smear or pregnancy results, you won't usually be told over the phone.

Whether you get your diagnosis immediately or after a while, make sure you take a friend with you. As I suggested in the chapter on examination, spend a few moments making contact with the consultant. Then you are ready to go on to discuss the diagnosis.

Diagnosis

Working together

Remember that the doctor's diagnosis is only an external comment on your health. It can be tempting to place all the responsibility on the doctor, to wait to be told what is the matter with you; but you don't have to hand over total control like this.

In fact, you will probably have thought about what might be the matter with you. Many women 'knew there was something wrong' – tiredness, feeling out of sorts, an awareness of 'lack of balance' as one woman described it, could have indicated that you were not well.

So maybe we can move towards a situation where patient and doctor can work together to arrive at a diagnosis. In many ways, we already do; the doctor asks you questions about your medical history, and you tell her/him about your symptoms. We all go to the diagnosis with some idea, right or wrong, of what we think is the matter.

Try taking things a stage further than this. Before you see your doctor, spend some time considering your body, becoming aware of any symptoms you have, and what feelings you have noticed. It could be that nothing comes to mind or else you might gradually become conscious of what is wrong with you. If you have had definite symptoms, such as vaginal discharge or bleeding, then try to remember when, how much and of what type; for example, do you bleed after intercourse? (many women do so without having cancer); is your vaginal discharge clear or coloured? Remember that you might have a tendency to think the worst about what is happening to you, and so try to be aware of when you are offering useful information – 'I've noticed that I have pain on intercourse, but only at certain times of the month' – and when you are simply panicking.

Then, when you are with the consultant, try asking whether the doctor would be interested in hearing your opinions about your condition. If your doctor is willing, tell her/him what feelings you have noticed, any symptoms you have identified, what your instincts tell you. If the doctor listens, s/he will learn a great deal, and may be able to make a more accurate diagnosis. You will have taken a part in what is happening, rather than simply waiting to be told what is the matter with you.

Questions and answers

At this point, the doctor will begin to discuss your diagnosis, hopefully in language you can understand. Do ask for explanations of terms that you are not familiar with. Maybe s/he will show you a photograph of your cervix, showing the normal and abnormal cells, or draw a diagram to demonstrate where the abnormality is and how far it has spread. This is the time to ask further questions. Remember that if you have just had your examination and are feeling a bit shaky, your friend can ask the questions for you. Some questions women asked were these:

> *What exactly did you find during the colposcopy?*
> *What was my repeat smear result?*
> *What did the punch/cone biopsy show?*
> *What grade of CIN do I have?*
> *How far has it spread?*
> *Can you tell me now whether my condition is cancerous or pre-cancerous?*

Remember to ask the doctor to explain again anything you don't understand. There may be pressure on her/him to complete your appointment quickly, because there are other people waiting, but for you this is an important opportunity to confer with a professional who knows your condition – so take it.

You may not only want to know about your CIN condition. It might be important for you and for your partner to know about any other conditions of your cervix. Even if no treatment is needed, there might be some sort of infection or virus that you should know about so that you can deal with it.

And as you will know from reading Chapter 9 on causes, it is important to know whether you have the wart virus. So further questions to ask are:

> *Did you notice any inflammation in my cervix? Do you know what might be causing this?*
> *Was there any vaginal discharge? Can you suggest what might be causing this?*
> *Did you find any evidence of a viral infection, particularly the wart virus?*

Possibilities

All clear

It is possible that after a preliminary positive smear result, a few months later you show no signs of abnormal cells. This is possibly the best news of all. It shows what has been suspected, and has been demonstrated by an American study of women with the condition: that it is reversible.[1]

However, you do need to look at what in your life made you vulnerable to developing the abnormal cells in the first place. If you do this – perhaps by reading the chapters in this book on causes and on prevention – you may find that in order to make yourself less vulnerable in the future, you need to change something about your life.

Infections and viruses

You probably will have been told by your GP about any infections or viruses you have. The consultant may add an extra comment about them, or suggest you have them treated if you aren't doing so already.

In particular, as I explain in the chapter on causes, a virus which causes genital warts in men has been suggested as playing a part in some cases of cervical cancer and CIN. This is, as I comment elsewhere in the book, not a clear-cut issue. But even if you do not consider the wart virus to be responsible for your cervical condition, your consultant may do, and so may want to tell you about that.

Cervical erosion

If the consultant notices that you have a cervical erosion, s/he may tell you this. Remember that, as explained in the chapter on Facts, this does not mean that your cervix is being eroded away – just that the softer, more vulnerable cervical cells are now exposed in your vagina.

CIN (Cervical intraepithelial neoplasia) or abnormal cell change

It is almost certain that your positive smear is due to a pre-cancerous condition of the cervix. So the likelihood is that the doctor will tell you that you have a CIN condition, grades 1, 2 or 3. This means, as we see in Chapter 8, that you have some cells on your cervix that are abnormal and treatable. You may not even need treatment, if the condition is in the early stages.

If this is your news, then the most logical thing for you to do is to jump up and down in the consulting room shouting for joy. For you are one of the majority of women in whom a pre-cancerous condition has been spotted in good time. And once you have treated the condition, you have a high chance of never being bothered with it again. That is the logic of the situation.

However, we are not logical beings. Straightforward as the medical facts are, we can still feel upset, frightened and angry. We have brains and emotions, and they get carried along too. So if you are diagnosed like this, and you still feel a bit weepy or at a loss, or if you are still worried about treatment or other people's reactions, you are perfectly normal – and you are not alone.

'After my colposcopy I was told: "the cells are abnormal, but don't worry." I didn't worry. I was concerned.' (Judith).

'I was clear from the start that it was never cancer. I think I coped well, but I did get down sometimes, for other reasons.' (Evelyn).

What if it is cancer?

Your doctor may tell you that you have cervical cancer. The thing to remember is that it is highly unlikely that you will die. The annual death rate from cervical cancer is 2,000 (as compared to 15,000 women a year who die of breast cancer). However remember that 85 per cent of women who have cervical cancer have never had a smear; of the 15 per cent left, most have only ever had one smear. The fact that you have, that your condition has been noticed through an examination, rather than left to become more advanced, means that you have more than a very good chance of total recovery. Mostly, nowadays, cancer does not kill.

I spoke in my interviews to three women who had had cervical cancer. They had all had hysterectomies, two had had radical radiotherapy. All three have now passed the five year 'all-clear' point, and I can testify that they are all energetic, powerful, vital women. These are some of the things they said to me:

'Since then, I've been on an assertiveness course for women. I've learned to ask for what I want.' (Sue).

'Yes, my life did change . . . I worry so much less now.' (Jane).

These women are not in any way saying that if you have cervical cancer then everything is fine. What they are saying is that it is not the end.

It is possible, at this point, that if you have had cancer diagnosed, you will need to supplement this book with other sources of information. You are travelling a different path from most of the women who have a positive smear. If you look in the Resource section of this book, you will find a full list of many of the support services for cancer, and a long list of books written especially for you and your problems and challenges.

Pregnancy

A few of the women I spoke to had been pregnant when they discovered that they had a cervical condition. A smear test is often routine in the first stages of pregnancy, and this can be the time that your cervical condition is first spotted.

This is a difficult situation and merits talking through carefully with your doctor. You can't have treatment while you are pregnant, and this may concern you.

Often there is no danger to yourself or your baby and an early case of CIN may well be left untreated until after you have given birth. If you went through the normal system, it is possible you would have to wait six months for treatment anyway, so you are in no worse a position.

If your condition is more serious, then you will need to take some informed decisions. Developing cervical cancer when pregnant is rare, so I am not going to dwell on it in too much detail. However you may have to face up to the fact that a normal pregnancy and cervical cancer are not easily compatible, and that you have to choose between them.

On the other hand, two of the women I talked to who had

cervical abnormality were advised to go through with their pregnancies and have a hysterectomy immediately afterwards. Your
doctor will be able to talk through with you exactly what your
decisions should be.

Match or mismatch?

Usually, your idea of what is wrong with you and the doctor's
diagnosis agree. You respect her/his professional ability and you
know in your heart that what s/he says is right, whether you like it
or not. It can sometimes happen though that your diagnosis and the
doctor's don't match. You feel your condition is not what s/he says
it is. Look at these feelings carefully. You may have been so upset
by the diagnosis that you are refusing to believe it. However if you
calmly and coolly believe that you are right and the diagnosis is
wrong, then this is an opportunity to look after yourself in the best
way possible. There are several things you can do about a mismatch
between your instincts and your doctor's diagnosis.

You might be tempted to ignore the diagnosis completely; this is
never a good thing to do. 'I thought – if I just go home, and not let
them touch me, then it will all go away.' (Sue). Fortunately, Sue
didn't just go home, and she did survive cervical cancer.

You can challenge your doctor. You can ask her/him to examine
you again and see if your condition is still the same. The condition
might have retreated, and before you progress to treatment, you
will want to be sure you really need it. Another option is to ask for a
second opinion, or change doctors completely. Heather was dis-
satisfied with her doctor's diagnosis that her cervical condition was
not serious and could be left untreated for six months. She went
back to the clinic with a friend, and demanded another smear. Her
condition had worsened; she then fought for, and received, laser
treatment.

Diagnosis – right and responsibility

The vast majority of diagnoses are correct – and in the over-
strained health service, we shouldn't let simple panic or distress
push us to illogical demands on the medical profession. However if

you do believe that your diagnosis is wrong, then to challenge it is your right – and your responsibility.

In the long term, after the positive smear diagnosis is in the past, you can learn from the whole experience to take notice of what your body is saying and begin to take responsibility for its health. You can become more conscious of when you are ill, and when you are truly well. You can begin to diagnose your own physical state, using the doctor to confirm or make more accurate what you have found out for yourself. Then you will have learned something, you will have increased your chances of health in the future. And in the interim you will be able to move on towards treatment and towards cure.

5

WHICH TREATMENT –
ALTERNATIVE WAYS

_____

All this aggressive treatment . . . isn't there a better way?
(Tracey)

Your condition has been diagnosed. All that remains is for you to have the condition 'zapped away' as one consultant put it. In fact, I don't think that it need be like this. I think that there is a case for stopping and thinking. The consultant has her/his own pattern of recommending treatment. S/he does it all in good faith, and is usually correct. Your view is a little different. Yours is the only case you have to think about at the moment. You have little professional expertise, but when the treatment is over, you are the person who has to live with the consequences. So stopping and thinking is often a good idea.

For there is a pattern, even in the early stages of CIN, of recommending strong, 'aggressive' treatment as a matter of course – laser, cone biopsy, cryosurgery. There is a temptation to 'zap and discharge' a patient, and in many cases this is the only alternative for doctors who are concerned that if they offer gentler forms of treatment the condition will spread or the patient simply never return for check-ups. With your awareness, and your concern for yourself, maybe you have other alternatives.

A word of warning is needed here. The more advanced your condition, the further along the scale of CIN-cancer you are, the less time you have to stop and think, and the more advisable standard treatment is. I am not suggesting (for those panicking medical professionals who think I am) that you go home and allow yourself to die of advanced invasive cancer with secondaries.

But in Britain today, we have a situation in which the waiting list for diagnosis, not to mention the treatment, is often of several months. This scandal can actually be quite good news for those of us who prefer to try gentler methods of treatment before agreeing to more aggressive methods such as laser. I would suggest that we could use this time to do something ourselves.

Many of the women I spoke to did this. Jane G. had laser treatment but supported it with homoeopathy for 'the anxiety, the bruising and the shock. When I went back, the surgeon commented on how well I'd healed.'

This chapter then, covers some alternative, less invasive approaches that you may choose to use yourself, particularly if you have CIN 1 and 2, before agreeing to hospital treatment. Remember that in such cases it can be better to go for the total health of the body rather than for the total destruction of a few rogue cells.

Treatment choices

Do nothing

This is not really a viable option. The particular circumstances that made you vulnerable to the cervical condition are probably still present, and unless something happens, the changing cells on your cervix will continue to change. So *never* ignore it. It won't go away.

Build health

You can try and prevent cervical conditions developing by being as healthy as you can be, and you can also support whatever treatment you receive in the same way. Building health won't suddenly create spontaneous remission of any disease you have – but it will allow you to get better more quickly, and it is something you can do all by yourself.

What should you be doing? Your aim is to become as healthy as you can in a fairly short time, without straining an already vulnerable system. There are several ways to build health, and many books on the subject and the chapter in this book on Prevention outlines some of the ways you can build health long-term.

Changes to diet can't be made overnight, but you can cut down on obviously harmful things such as too much fat or sugar. If you are on drugs or tranquillizers, try to cut down, though do check with your doctor first that this will be appropriate.

It is also advisable, particularly if you are going to have a general anaesthetic, to work on improving your lung power. Don't suddenly leap into an intensive jogging programme when you haven't even run for a bus for the last two years. Take regular, gentle exercise; frenetic activity such as looking after two under-fives doesn't count, by the way! Try swimming as one woman did: 'to feel my body was participating in getting more healthy.' Relax for a few minutes several times a day. Do lots of things you enjoy and that make you feel good.

Vitamins and minerals

There are three dietary elements that are often absent in women with cervical cancer and CIN. Recent work done in America has suggested that taking regular doses of these in early cases of cervical abnormality may prove useful. They can be obtained by making sure your diet includes those foods which contain them, or by taking synthetic vitamin and mineral supplements, available from any good chemist or health food store.

Vitamin C, found in citrus fruits and uncooked vegetables, is a water-soluble vitamin which passes out of your system through your urine if you take too much. Try to eat more of these foods, and supplement your diet with vitamin C tablets; 100 mg is the recommended daily amount, though some doctors say that 10 g is standard cancer therapy. It is not a case of more is better though; if you overdose on vitamin C, you may find yourself with diarrhoea.

Folic acid, is found in yeast, wheatgerm, nuts and pulses. It can also be taken as a supplement, and one recommended dose is 10 mg a day. Oral contraceptives can create folic acid deficiency, so if you are on the Pill you might like to try taking a supplement, although again, too much is not a good idea.

Beta carotene, found particularly in carrots, green leafy vegetables, apricots and peaches, is another possible treatment. One woman started drinking carrot juice from the time of her smear up to the time of her laser treatment – and claims it improved her eyesight too. There is a danger of overdosing however, so as a general rule, two glasses a day will do. Large doses of synthetic beta carotene or vitamin A need to be taken under supervision, though the amounts included in most multivitamin pills are safe – as long as you stick to the recommended dosage.

Barrier contraception

The chapter on Causes explains how using barrier contraception may decrease vulnerability in your cervix. Using a barrier method is not only a good way to prevent, but also to treat your condition. In an American study[2] of 135 women with abnormal cervical cells, 133 of them got better spontaneously simply by their partner using a condom over a period of several months. This amazingly simple and trouble-free way of curing cervical problems seems to have been largely ignored by medical professionals in the West and I do wonder why; perhaps they are frightened it won't work, or perhaps it just seems too easy. It also places the control back in the patient's hands, which is sometimes hard for doctors to handle.

Naturally, I am not suggesting that using barrier contraception will cure all CIN conditions. Nor would I suggest that using a condom and never going back for a repeat smear is the answer. Changing to barrier methods might anyway be difficult for you and your partner, for a number of reasons, but do look carefully at the advantages.

If you have a positive smear, try using a barrier method of contraception immediately. If you have been told simply to come back for a repeat smear, use it until then. If you have a more severe condition on the CIN grade, then in the intervals between the news and the diagnosis and treatment, try using a barrier method. During further examination, a repeat smear may well reveal that your condition has now cleared up.

If your condition proves to need further treatment, you have lost nothing at all by using barrier contraception. And you can choose to have that treatment just as before. If you have in fact cured yourself, then congratulations. You've avoided the upset to your body of further treatment. Tell your consultant and everyone else about your success in a loud voice. A further reason for using contraception (whether it be barrier contraception or another method) once you have had a positive smear, is that it is vitally important not to get pregnant while you are waiting for treatment. Your being pregnant may confuse any diagnosis, and you can't have treatment while you are pregnant.

Remember that after you have a clear result, you need to consider the issues involved before deciding whether to stop using barrier contraception.

Clearing up infections

Infections can mask other conditions of the cervix, so you should get them cleared up as soon as you can. You can ask your doctor for treatment, if s/he hasn't already suggested this. There is a range of strong antibiotics to treat most vaginal infections, and they are often quick and effective. You may want to think carefully before taking antibiotics, however, because they do lower your immunity to infection and they can stay in your bloodstream for a long time afterwards. Depending on what your particular infection is, there are sometimes more natural alternatives available; the leaflets, books and contacts in the Resource section will give you further help with this.

Clearing up viruses

The viruses that are most linked with CIN are herpes and wart virus. So along with any treatment that takes care of CIN conditions you need also to clear these up if you have them. Usually your doctor will have spotted their existence on the first smear and offered you treatment. If not, the consultant may mention them during your colposcopy. If you know you have either of these viruses and doctors do not mention treating them, then mention it yourself. Remember that if you are to stay virus-free, both you and your partner may need to be treated.

Both conditions can clear up spontaneously and if you are healthy and stress-free, then this is more likely to happen. However it is more probable that you need to see your doctor or attend a special clinic at the hospital in order to get treatment. Don't be put off by the fact that the special clinic is for sexually transmitted diseases – this very fact means that the staff may well be more at ease with your condition than your family doctor is.

Herpes. Things to do for yourself are: wash often and gently, avoiding soap; do not wear anything that can irritate the herpes such as tight briefs or nylon. Increase your zinc intake with a mineral supplement, taking care not to exceed the recommended amount. If the herpes is painful, take pain-killers. Current orthodox treatment offered by hospitals includes drugs that seem to have good results, and antiseptic creams. It's very important not to reinfect yourself or your partner, so keep towels and clothes separate while you have an attack. For further information on herpes treatment and support, see the Resource section.

Wart virus. Unfortunately for us and our partners, conventional treatment for genital warts can be lengthy and painful. One doctor suggested to me that the treatment may actually be more traumatic than the symptoms! Furthermore, many doctors are so convinced of the unlikelihood of infection that they do not even suggest that both partners be treated. If you do want treatment, however, there are a variety of remedies available and what you are offered will depend on where you attend and what your condition is: one treatment uses chemicals to burn away the warts, a process which takes two to three weeks. In cauterization the warts are destroyed by the application of heat or liquid nitrogen and this is usually done under anaesthetic. If you can have a local anaesthetic, do so, but some warts can be so deep inside the vagina that you need to have a general anaesthetic for treatment.

Laser treatment also destroys cervical warts, and a further possibility is to have them removed surgically. There is a new experimental drug called Immunovir which is currently being tested to support the other methods; as yet there are no positive results.

One suggested self-treatment for warts is a homoeopathic remedy, Thuja, 6 potency, tablets taken regularly over a period of four to six weeks. Thuja tincture can also be painted on the warts. A good homoeopathic chemist can supply both and advise you on usage.

For further information and support, see the Resource section.

Treating cervical erosion

Cervical erosion itself is not harmful, and many doctors don't think it necessary to treat it. If you have an abnormal smear, then this indicates that treatment is needed. Orthodox treatment for CIN which involves burning or freezing will do this, but if you are not having this, perhaps because you are coming back for a repeat smear, you or your doctor might decide that it is worth treating any discharge with sulfa cream which is inserted in the vagina. Remember that if the erosion is harmless – that is if you get a negative result on your smear – it is usually accepted that there is no need to treat it.

Complementary medicine

There are many forms of complementary medicine. The doctors who practise them work mostly outside the National Health Service and you have to pay to consult them. There is also the problem of standards; for in some areas of medicine anyone can set up as a practitioner, even without training. Some women I spoke to reported negative experiences with complementary treatments: 'I wasn't all that convinced by it.' (Emma); while some reported positive experiences: 'My homoeopath was marvellous and very supportive of my decision to have laser treatment.' (Jane G.).

The Institute of Complementary Medicine and the organization New Approaches to Cancer both offer guidelines to recommended practitioners. It is worth contacting them if you want to step outside mainstream medicine.

Most of these complementary approaches do not attempt to cure your condition, be it an infection, CIN, or cancer, and will only aim to improve your general health. Most of them suggest you use their services alongside the treatment suggested by your consultant.

Some useful complementary approaches are these:

Reflexology. Your current state of health can be revealed by an examination of your feet. Foot massage can stimulate your immune system to help you fight disease.

Iridology. The iris of the eye is studied and your current general health diagnosed. Practitioners usually offer no treatment but will probably make some recommendations about your diet and life-style.

Massage. There are nearly as many forms of massage as there are bodies to be massaged. Some masseurs claim to heal by touch, others to stimulate energy centres in the body so that your immune system works harder. As long as you feel comfortable with the masseur, just being relaxed will strengthen you.

Meditation. Again, there are many schools. If you feel that you are stressed and need to relax, this can be helpful. You don't always need to take a philosophy on board in order to do it.

Dietary therapies. Alterations to your diet can help get rid of harmful waste products and boost your immune system. Beware of too strict a diet, because it can lower your energy reserves.

Acupuncture. Pressure and needle-puncture are used to release energy along 'channels' in the body. Acupuncturists sometimes offer advice on life-styles too.

Homoeopathy. The purpose is to build health rather than to treat symptoms. One homoeopath I spoke to said he would not treat cervical conditions directly; another said he would only treat any bruising or emotional upset caused by orthodox treatment.

Visualization. Some therapists believe that by visualizing the disease, you can control it. Work done with cancer patients by the

Simontons in the USA over the last decade is now famous, although the Simontons themselves are rethinking their approach.

Emotional therapies.   Co-counselling provides a self-help tool to release emotion safely (and cheaply). If you feel that your recovery would be helped by being able to express your emotions more fully, this may be for you. Other forms of psychotherapy and counselling usually involve working under the guidance of another person to build your mental and emotional resources and resolve past traumas in your life. They usually entail detailed change of your ways of thinking, and might therefore be both too long-term and too expensive to consider. Some short-term therapies, such as Neuro-Linguistic Programming have a good record of quick and effective work with illness.

The Bristol Cancer Help Centre provides a rounded approach to cancer care based on a variety of alternative methods. You can spend a day or a week there, depending on your needs, learning about some of the approaches mentioned here. Bristol will accept patients who have CIN, though the treatment and consultations are aimed at the cancer sufferer. The service is private and quite costly and the Centre has been criticized for having no medical effect on the disease. However, the Centre and its staff are impressive: effective, kind and supportive. Many of its patients report long-term improvement, and visiting the Centre may well change the quality of your life for the better.

The above notes on approaches are very brief: if you want further information, contact one of the referral organizations mentioned in the Resource section of this book.

Alternative approaches – yes or no?

As to the question of whether to try any of the approaches mentioned in this chapter, there are two issues to consider: first you need to decide whether to try them, and then you need to decide whether to try to cure yourself through them. The first issue seems pretty clear cut – unless you overdose on vitamins or choose a totally incompetent therapist, you are unlikely to do yourself any harm by attempting the alternative methods. Some of them – like taking exercise or practising relaxation – can immeasurably improve the quality of your life; you might find, as some women did, that having a positive smear was the starting point of a healthier, happier lifestyle.

To rely on these approaches alone to cure you is an altogether different matter. In this case you have to consider how serious your condition is, how much time you have, and how important it is to you not to be treated by conventional methods. Here a useful guideline seems to be that mentioned earlier – if you have time between diagnosis and orthodox treatment, use it, and you may well heal yourself. If you have no time, then think carefully before saying no to what is often a totally effective cure.

6

WHICH TREATMENT – ORTHODOX WAYS

> They don't usually let you choose . . . I just kept going
> until they did. (Lily)

We look now at the treatments you can expect to be offered in a
hospital. They all involve removing the abnormal cells in some way
– by burning, freezing or cutting.

As mentioned before, there is a general disadvantage in all of
these; they damage the body and create distress. 'Having third
degree burns on your cervix takes a bit of getting over', as one
woman put it. Also, some of the treatments involved have to be
administered under general anaesthetic, which carries its own
risks. Jane G., a singer, refused to have a cone biopsy because she
didn't want to have a general anaesthetic, since it involves the
insertion into the throat of a ventilation tube. She changed doctors
and received laser treatment, which in her case cleared the abnormal cells and didn't entail a general anaesthetic. Although it is very
rare to have a positive smear during pregnancy, if you do, it is
particularly important to think through the alternatives when you
have two lives to look after.

You should remember that although doctors usually know their
job, they also have their likes and dislikes. One consultant will use
freezing, another favour surgery, while a third may be in the habit
of using laser to treat young women and cone biopsy to treat older
women. They deal with hundreds of women a week and develop
patterns of treatment. You can suggest a more informed alternative
based on the needs of your life once you know what options are
available.

You can then perhaps negotiate with your doctor to have a

different form of treatment, or change doctors to get what you want. But if two doctors in a row say that you really must have one particular form of treatment, think very carefully before you argue. One may be biased, but two is more than a coincidence.

Treatments – a quick tour

How do you choose? What follows is a brief outline of the various treatments and their advantages and disadvantages. You can use this as a quick guideline when comparing different treatments. Later in this chapter are full descriptions of what each involves. It is important to keep things in perspective. Reading about hysterectomy here doesn't mean you are going to have to have one; few women do.

Laser is an infra-red beam that vaporizes abnormal cells. It is usually used in CIN cases and is normally carried out in Out-patients under local anaesthetic. The after-effects are usually minimal and its ease and speed of treatment have made it very popular.

Cryocautery. Liquid nitrogen is applied in order to destroy the cells. It is usually used to treat CIN 1 or 2 and is done in Out-patients. It is cheaper than a laser, so more hospitals offer it.

Cold coagulation. This is used less often than other methods. It is actually a heat treatment similar to hot wire cautery and diathermy but it is used when the condition is not so severe. It is also a cheaper form of treatment, so you could find your hospital offers it, rather than the more expensive laser.

Hot wire cautery and diathermy. In these methods, the abnormal cells are burnt away by wire or electrodes. They are used when CIN is severe or can't be reached by a laser, and since they are done under general anaesthetic, they often involve an overnight stay in hospital. The after-effects of these treatments are similar to those with laser, but having a general anaesthetic can affect you for some time.

Cone or cylinder biopsy. This is surgical removal of a cone- (or cylinder-) shaped piece of the cervix. It is done under general anaesthetic and you will probably have to spend a few days in hospital. It is used in more advanced forms of CIN, particularly when other forms of treatment could not reach abnormal cells that have developed far up the cervix. It is also sometimes used to diagnose cancer; the piece removed can be tested in the laboratory to find out whether it is malignant and how far the malignancy has spread.

Hysterectomy is the removal of the womb, sometimes along with the ovaries and part of the vagina and lymph nodes. When cancer has spread, hysterectomy is almost always carried out, but it may also be offered if you are past child-bearing age, even if your condition is not very serious. So check carefully what your options are before agreeing to the operation. It takes several days in hospital and weeks of recovery, and you must also consider the emotional effects of losing your womb. However, if the cancer is truly massive, then hysterectomy may be the best option.

Radiotherapy. Radiation treatment used to kill cancer, or to remove any last traces of cancer after a hysterectomy. The treatment can consist of daily doses under a machine for several weeks, or in the vagina for twenty-four hours. There are side effects, though these are often over-dramatized. It is usually only recommended when cancer is present and you need it in order to survive.

Chemotherapy. Injected drugs are used along with surgery. This is rarely used with cervical conditions. It has all the effects (and most of the side effects) of radiotherapy.

Negotiating treatment with the doctor

When will you discuss treatment with your doctor? It will almost certainly be when the consultant diagnoses you, after the colposcopy or when the results of the biopsy or cone biopsy come back. The doctor will tell you what s/he wants to do (and when). So it is wise when going for your diagnosis to be prepared to discuss treatment at the same time. You might react strongly to your doctor's suggestions of treatment, just as you can react strongly to her/his diagnosis. Everything suggested in the chapters on examination and diagnosis applies here too; you do have the right to discuss treatment with your consultant, even if you don't get the response you want.

Whatever you feel, you will probably want to begin by asking your doctor some questions, and these are some of the questions that women I talked to asked:

> *What treatment do you think would be best for me?*
> *Why are you choosing this sort of treatment?*
> *What will be the after effects of this treatment (on my ability to have children, make love, etc)?*
> *Will my treatment mean my changing methods of contraception (will I have to have my I U C D removed)?*
> *What would be the position if I wanted to have . . . (any other form of treatment than the one the doctor has mentioned)?*
> *Why would you not recommend this?*
> *I am concerned about these things; could I talk them through with you?*
> *When would you treat me?*
> *Will I be an out-patient? (If so, when, for how long?)*
> *Will I be an in-patient? (If so, when, for how long?)*

Discussing these things will give you some idea of the way the consultant is thinking. His/her answers may satisfy you and make you feel happier about what is happening. The final few questions will also give you an idea of that particular hospital's waiting list, and the length of your own treatment (vital points when arranging child care).

When you have heard the doctor's answers, you may also wish to negotiate with him/her on a number of things. Firstly, you might want to delay treatment in case the condition clears up. It is rarely possible to speed treatment up. Secondly, you might want to opt for another form of treatment, and if so arrange for it to be done in another hospital. Or perhaps you want him/her to refer you for another form of treatment at another hospital.

Your doctor will react in one of a number of ways. S/he may

agree to what you suggest, in which case you have got what you wanted, secure in the knowledge that your doctor believes it is medically sound.

Your doctor may disagree, and refuse to give you the treatment you have requested. If so, do not agree right away to his/her suggestions without taking time to think. If you are concerned, go home and think through the whole issue of treatment. Talk about it with people close to you, or with professionals if you need to. Think about just what you would prefer your treatment to be. For many of us, particularly with minor conditions, the decision is easily made. If your condition is more serious, think more carefully about which option to go for.

Treatment choice – Out-patients

Laser treatment, cryocautery or cold coagulation are the most likely possibilities for out-patient treatment, which is usually easier and less trouble. Some of the women I talked to had gone into hospital overnight for these treatments, because for one reason or another they had needed a general anaesthetic, but usually it is a one-day affair.

You will be asked to bring a friend or partner. You may want to read over the comments in the chapters on Examination and Building Your Own Support System to help you think through the issues surrounding this. All the things I said there apply again. Also remember to book child care or time off from work – and to arrange your appointment so that it doesn't clash with your period.

If you have an IUCD, you may have been told that it has to be removed during your treatment. You will therefore need to start using another method of contraception, and this may entail some thinking ahead – for example if you want to start taking the Pill.

Take with you your own sanitary towel and perhaps some pain-killers in case you need them. One woman reported taking a homoeopathic liquid called The Rescue Remedy (for shock and trauma) immediately after her treatment, and said she felt much better within minutes.

At the hospital

After you have reached the hospital and are checked in and waiting, try preparing for what is going to happen by relaxing. This may sound difficult, for you are facing an operation, even though it is minor. But the more you relax, the less of a jolt to your system the treatment will be. As mentioned before, it is also good to give and receive support with other women in the waiting-room.

The treatment room will be very similar to the room in which you had your examination. Most hospitals nowadays allow you to bring your friend or partner in with you, so that you have someone to hold your hand. If your hospital doesn't suggest your friend comes in with you, mention it anyway; they might say yes if you ask.

Remembering as always to take your briefs with you, you then lie down on an examination couch with your legs on supports as before. It is at this point that your IUCD, if you have one, will be removed. This can come as a great shock if you are not expecting it: 'Naughty that, not telling you,' was Rosemary's comment. Some consultants will replace your IUCD after treatment, if they are confident that this will not increase your risk of infection.

Treatment – laser, cryosurgery, cold coagulation

If you are having laser treatment, the doctor will as usual place a speculum in your vagina and open it. Then s/he will give you a local anaesthetic, which is an injection into your cervix. Some women complained that this was actually the most painful part of the whole process. Next, as the anaesthetic begins to take effect, the consultant will dab solution on your cervix as before, to show up the abnormal areas.

Then s/he will position the equipment – laser, cryosurgery machine or cold coagulator, at the entrance to your vagina. You probably won't see the equipment as you will be lying flat, although you may hear it; if you are having laser treatment, it 'makes a noise like a Hoover', as Julia said. The doctor will direct the machine carefully on to the abnormal cells. Treatment will take up to half an hour; the consultant will take his/her time so that s/he is sure that all the abnormal cells have been eradicated.

Does it hurt? As always this depends on what treatment you are having, how tense you are and how skilful the doctor is. Women I spoke to reported every kind of reaction from 'painless and very quick' (Rosemary) through 'a mild period pain' (Mary), to 'a very bad ache across your tummy' (Anna). Many hospitals will give you pain-killers if you need them, but it is always wise to bring your own.

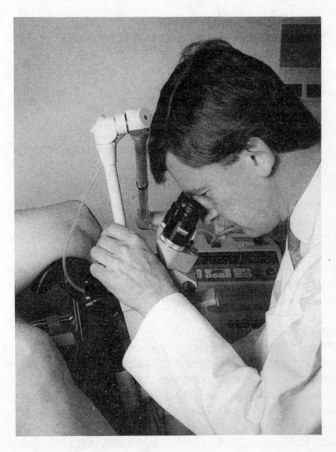

Figure 5. A laser machine in use.

How you react when it is happening also depends on many things. Mary reported that she 'lost her centre of gravity', while Emma found it 'a strong space, very relaxed . . . my partner was with me.' You can feel quite panicky, or know that at last you are being cured.

Afterwards, most hospitals provide a room where you can lie down and recover after the treatment. By this time, you will have put your briefs back on, with the sanitary towel. If you can, relax and rest until you feel better, and perhaps talk to your partner or friend about how you felt and what it was like. You may not want to talk at all, but just take time to assimilate what has happened in your own way.

If possible, have a cup of something hot before going to collect the medicine that you need to take with you for afterwards. This medicine will probably be antiseptic cream, although sometimes an antibiotic is prescribed to stop your wound becoming infected.

Afterwards – physical reactions

Women react very differently to these cervical treatments. Some take them in their stride; for many there is a 'kickback', as Rosemary described it.

The physical side-effects can be quite unexpected. I found that few hospitals think to warn patients sufficiently of what to expect, probably in order not to scare them. This is important, but just as important is knowing what might happen.

All the treatments given in Out-patients have side effects of one sort or another. Many women said they felt tired and weepy: 'I tried to go shopping just afterwards, but it was a mistake,' said Rosemary.

Another unexpected problem can be having to insert vaginal cream to heal the area that has been treated. You will need to insert an applicator containing the cream into your vagina – and this is usually best done lying on your back or your side. Some women find this difficult, others find it surprisingly funny: 'On my back, legs apart, and with one foot jammed up against the bathroom door because it doesn't have a lock on it,' was one woman's hilarious description.

You will probably have discharge whichever treatment you had: 'Smelly watery black bits,' as Julie described it; 'Bits of floating mushroom,' as Linda said. It's best to wear a sanitary towel rather than tampons for about four weeks to avoid the risk of infection. Be prepared too for bleeding which lasts much longer than you expect it to. As you leave after treatment ask your consultant for some indication of how long this bleeding might last. Almost every woman I spoke to reported bleeding which was heavier or longer than she expected. If you become anxious at any time after your treatment, go, as I did, to your GP. Some hospitals provide a number to ring if you are worried – and of course if the problem is really serious, you can go to Out-patients.

The hospital will probably advise you not to make love for a while after the treatment. Times given vary widely, and it is a temptation to make love when you feel like it. The comfort of making love must surely be an aid to convalescence, though doing so too early increases the risk of infection. It is best to wait at least two weeks after your treatment.

Long term side effects of these treatments seem to be very few: they don't affect your ability to have children or to enjoy love-making. Some women complain of spotting or light bleeding for a long time afterwards, but in general the healing is clear and clean.

Afterwards – emotional reactions

The emotional reactions to cervical treatment may be less notice-able – or last far longer. Having treatment on your cervix that attacks and yet cures it is a strange experience. It can make you feel scared, angry, or 'very sad' as Rosemary said. More than one woman commented on the feeling of being penetrated, and the contradiction between wanting to pull away and wanting to be cured. Emma summed it up when she said: 'You feel it coming into you. You feel you need to protect yourself, yet you know you have to keep still if it's going to work.'

However many women reported feeling elated after the treat-ment. They knew that the problem was now more than likely gone for ever. There can be a sense of 'triumph – I did it!' as one woman reported. Most women said they felt more negative emotions –

fear, for example – before the operation, than after. Once it is over, you will quite possibly have a sense of being cured both physically and emotionally.

Treatment choice – In-patient

You may be wary of going into hospital, particularly if you've never done so before. On a practical level, however, there is often very little difference between this and out-patient treatment; it just takes more time, that's all.

All of the treatments we now look at involve a general anaesthetic – although some of the women I talked to had also had a general anaesthetic for laser treatment. This usually means an overnight stay in hospital, with all that that involves. A word of warning – if you develop a streaming cold just before the operation, don't even bother going to the hospital, as it is very unlikely they will operate. Ring them the day before, explain the situation and ask their advice.

When you arrive at the hospital, the receptionist will usually tell you which ward to report to, and when you get there a nurse will show you to a bed. The waiting, sometimes throughout that day until your operation the next morning, is often the worst. Take lots of reading (or knitting) with you and welcome visitors with open arms – you can get very bored.

The day will probably be full, however, as doctors examine you again, take a full medical history, a blood sample and check your lungs and blood pressure. Usually a junior doctor will see you to check the details, and the anaesthetist will visit you to check any problems with the anaesthetic. Occasionally the consultant who will do the operation will also call in to see you.

The night before the operation, don't be surprised if you can't get to sleep; you're in an unfamiliar place and possibly worried about tomorrow. The nurses may offer you sleeping tablets, or you may prefer to take a herbal or calcium sleeping remedy which will leave your body feeling more alert and ready to cope with the operation; some women said they used these and found them less 'drugging' than the hospital's alternative.

You won't be allowed anything to eat on the morning of the

operation, and you will be asked to bathe or shower and change into theatre clothes, a gown and cap. You'll sometimes be asked to remove your jewellery, and if you don't want to take your wedding ring off, this can usually be taped to your hand.

You will be asked to sign a consent form, saying that you understand what is going to happen and agree to it. Make very sure you get this explained to you – and that you do agree. Viki refused to sign a form saying that if the surgeon found cancer cells, he could perform a hysterectomy while she was on the operating table. She preferred to wait and talk it through with him after the operation rather than agree to it in advance.

You will probably then be given a pre-medication. It is usually given to calm you down, and reduce your saliva, which can make your mouth too slippery for the anaesthetist to cope with. You can add to the calming effect of the pre-med by using your own ways of relaxing – perhaps taking deep regular breaths, or remembering a time when you were particularly calm and strong within yourself.

When you are taken from the ward, you will be checked to make sure you are the right patient – you don't want to have the wrong operation done! In the ante-room to the theatre, the anaesthetist will inject the back of your hand with an anaesthetic solution. I remember my anaesthetist had a student with him, and I lost consciousness to the refrain of 'In that vein – not that one, that one . . .'

When you wake from the anaesthetic, you will have a dull ache in your stomach, and someone will have given you a sanitary towel (although more than likely not the briefs, so it will stick to the inside of your leg in a most off-putting manner).

As you wake, you will possibly be offered water to drink or ice to suck, and left to recover. This can take a few hours, or overnight, depending on the operation you've had, and you can expect to be very sleepy as a result of the drugs.

In some hospitals, women go home the same day, but in most, they stay in another night and are discharged after the consultant has seen them the next morning. Particularly with a cone biopsy, you can be asked to stay a day or two until you feel really better. The hospital will almost certainly give you antibiotics to help the

The cone removed

The raw area covered

Figure 6. Cone biopsy. A cone-shaped wedge of tissue is removed from the cervix.

healing process, and full instructions on how and when to take these.

Diathermy/hot wire cautery

The diathermy or hot wire operation itself is very similar to laser treatment. It's usually used when the CIN has spread far into your cervix and cannot quite be reached by laser. Diathermy penetrates more deeply into the cervix. Of course, you will know nothing about it, as the consultant uses the heat treatment only after you are deeply asleep from the anaesthetic.

Cone/cylinder biopsy

Another way of dealing with far-reaching CIN is a cone or cylinder biopsy. It is usually performed on older women, particularly on those who have finished having a family. The doctor may also use the operation to investigate your cervix (see p. 18), and make quite certain that there are no malignant cells. This is done by taking away skin to quite a deep level for later examination in the same way as in a punch biopsy. In a cone biopsy, a triangular wedge of the cervix is removed; in a cylinder biopsy it is a section shaped like a cylinder.

During the operation the surgeon will cut out the affected cells with a scalpel, in a cone or cylinder shape, and then cauterize the cervix to stop it bleeding. Recently, some operations have been done by laser. As always, antiseptic cream is applied. Soluble stitches or injections are given to stop you bleeding too much, and then your vagina is usually packed with fine gauze soaked in cream.

After the operation you will be kept in bed for about twenty-four hours. It is likely that you will be uncomfortable: 'It brings water to your eyes' (Lily), but the discomfort eases after the gauze is taken out. Sometimes you have to have a catheter inserted to allow you to pass water.

Afterwards – physical reactions

The after-effects of diathermy and hot wire treatment are the same as other heat-treatments like laser. Discharge and bleeding can last for a long time. I bled for five weeks, and on the fifth week dropped a blood clot that terrified me – although I then learned from my doctor that this is perfectly normal and is caused by the scab dropping off the cervical wound. In addition, the antibiotics I was given made me nauseous all the time.

The long-term physical effects of diathermy/hot-wire are usually the same as Out-patient treatments – normally none. The after-effects of a cone biopsy are usually bleeding problems. This is why the hospital suggests you stay in for a day or two after the operation, so that if serious bleeding starts they can treat you. You will continue to bleed for some time and should take it very easy while you convalesce – though Evelyn discharged herself from hospital the day after her operation and went straight to a weekend course.

It is probably quite unwise to begin love-making before at least six weeks have passed, to give your cervix time to heal, although you can ask your consultant about this. Bleeding might start again, or an infection take hold, and you are very vulnerable at this time.

The long-term effects of a cone biopsy can vary. Rachel's cervix closed together after her operation, and she had to have a second one to open it again. If this happens, your periods may stop (although you have to check that you aren't pregnant) and this can lead to complications. There is also a slight chance that having a cone biopsy, which takes away the tip of the cervix, could affect your ability to have children. The doctor will have thought of this, and may fight shy of suggesting this treatment to women who have not yet completed their family. But at least one childless woman I talked to was recommended a cone biopsy, which she refused.

As both of these treatments involve general anaesthetic, you may feel the after-effects of this too. It could take you days to feel really alert, depending on just how the antibiotics affect you and the amount of anaesthetic and pre-medication you've had. Remember that they are meant to slow down your nervous system and this is exactly what they do. Some women bounce straight back; some take a weekend of being sleepy and weepy before going back to work. After a cone biopsy take a few days convalescence if this is possible; your doctor will probably tell you how long to rest for.

Afterwards – emotional reactions

In some ways, in-patient operations can leave you less emotional than out-patient operations. You aren't left with the memories of having things done to you, and you don't need to cope with 'pulling yourself together' directly afterwards in order to go home.

On the other hand, these operations take a much bigger chunk out of your life. You may be out of action for a while, and you will be away from your home base at least overnight. Also, you are on your own, negotiating the hospital routine and the discomfort of the operation, without a friend or partner to hold your hand.

When you come out of hospital, try to make sure there is someone at home to be with you, at least overnight. One woman said, 'My partner picked me up from the hospital, brought me home and then went off on a golfing weekend. Even though I encouraged him to go, I still never quite forgave him.'

Expect to feel a bit odd for a while, particularly if you've had a cone biopsy and have been under general anaesthetic for longer. Take your support where you can, and give yourself time to get over things, physically and emotionally: 'I went straight from my cone biopsy off to a group of friends,' said one woman, 'and lapped up all the sympathy and looking-after I got!'

Treatment choice – radical methods

Radical treatments tend to be the treatments that make us scared – hysterectomy, radiotherapy, chemotherapy. There are lots of horror stories about things that go wrong, and how awful it can all be.

Mostly these treatments are used to cure cancer – although in the case of hysterectomy, it could be for a persistent pre-cancer or for treating other gynaecological problems at the same time.

If your doctor has said that you need to have one of these treatments, then you can choose not to have it. But as I said before, it is usually better, in these serious cases, to agree to the treatment. Supplement what is happening to you with your own ways of getting yourself better.

Build your health, physically and emotionally, and use all the resources you have – people, information, spiritual beliefs – to make the experience as positive as you can. Because this is a book about the whole experience of positive smear, and because radical treatments are called for in only a very small proportion of cases, I am only outlining what happens. At the back of the book you will find suggestions for reading matter in the form of specialist leaflets and books as well as the addresses of support groups and counselling services. Use them as starting points to get your own support system together.

There are two particular areas where you are likely to feel vulnerable. If you have gone from one examination to another, hoping for good news and always getting bad news, you may, like Sue did, 'feel my optimism waning.' If you know you have invasive cancer, you may be scared you are going to die. This is unlikely, but it is a fear you will naturally face, and you can find other people uneasy with it. Relatives and friends may be unable to talk to you because they fear the worst, and your partner may have emotions of his own to cope with.

Also, the thought of losing your ability to bear children can create strong emotion for you. If you are not yet past the age where you could have children, it may make you feel sad and as if you have lost something. As one woman said about her hysterectomy: 'It's not a form of contraception I'd recommend.'

There are support groups in most areas of the country where you can talk to women who have had a hysterectomy, get support from them and discuss your problems. Also, it's likely that the hospital you go to will offer you some counselling both before and after your hysterectomy. 'I cried a lot in hospital,' said Diana, 'away from the children in privacy. It's my way of coping with it.'

Final checks

It is likely that just before you have your treatment, your doctor
will want to have a final check to see how far the cancer has spread.

The first possibility is dilation and curettage (D&C). Note that in
some Health Authorities, this is regular examination procedure for
any abnormal smear (see page 18) so if your hospital chooses to do
one, this does not necessarily mean that you have cancer.

In a D&C, the cervical canal is dilated, a small probe is used to
examine your womb, and then the womb is scraped with a long,
thin instrument. The cervix is painted with iodine, and any areas
that do not stain are biopsied. The scraping and the biopsies are
examined to check for abnormality or invasive cancer. The procedure for this is the same as for any operation under general
anaesthetic, so re-read the section on in-patient preparation and
recovery. You might need to stay in hospital for a few days, then go
back later for your results.

A further check is a kidney scan (IVU or IVP) to check that the
cancer has not spread to your kidney system. This is rarely the case,
but if so, it does mean you are seriously ill. You will have a dye
injected in a vein, probably your arm. It goes through your
bloodstream and ends up in your kidneys, bladder and urethra.
You may feel a slight burning, but this soon passes, and then the
kidney X-ray will be taken.

Another type of scan that may be done is a Pelvic CT or CAT
scan. A complete picture of your womb and the organs around it is
taken by several small X-rays that are collected by computer and
displayed on to a TV screen. You will be asked to drink a special
liquid, a tampon will be put into your vagina, and a liquid inserted
into your anus. This allows your entire pelvis to be X-rayed
effectively.

Another type of scan is the ultrasound scan. For this you will first
be asked to drink lots of liquid to get a full bladder. My own
experience of this is that there are better ways of spending an
afternoon than lying on a couch being examined while your only
desire in the world is to have a pee. A gel is spread over the surface
of your abdomen and then a microphone is pressed down upon it.
This sends silent sound waves rippling through your full bladder.

The echoes of these sound waves are collected and converted by computer to make a picture that the doctor can examine.

A final test that might be done is a lymphogram, which checks whether your lymph system has been affected. Dye is injected into your feet, and will then pass through the lymph system up to your pelvis. An X-ray shows the doctor how the dye is passing through the system, and where any problems lie. The whole process takes a few hours, and will have the interesting side effect of your skin and urine turning a green colour.

Figure 7. Having an ultrasound scan at the Cromwell Hospital.

Hysterectomy

There are various kinds of hysterectomy, depending on just what is being taken away. A total hysterectomy is usually performed on women with earlier forms of cancer. This means that both the uterus and the cervix are removed, though not always the ovaries. In the case of younger women especially, the ovaries are usually left intact in order to avoid early menopausal symptoms. If more of your pelvis has been affected by the cancer, then your lymph glands might also be removed. Ask your consultant to explain to you exactly how s/he has planned your operation and what s/he needs to remove.

Although the operation is sometimes done through the vagina, it is more commonly performed by abdominal incision, a horizontal cut being made above your pubic hair; the scar usually heals well and is almost invisible. The alternative is a downwards cut, and you should check which your surgeon is doing. Sometimes a downwards cut cannot be avoided, but if possible ask if you can have the horizontal one – it's neater.

The preparations for a hysterectomy are the same as for any of the other operations mentioned in this book, except that you will be given a suppository to empty your bowels, and a section at the top of your pubic hair will be shaved off. It does grow back!

When you go for your operation, you will usually be given the

Figure 8. The extent of total hysterectomy.

anaesthetic in the back of your hand, as described earlier. Very occasionally you will be given an epidural, which means that the anaesthetic is injected into your spinal cord. This is similar to the anaesthetic administered to women when giving birth and it numbs the whole area below the point where the injection is given.

The operation itself usually takes about an hour. After your womb has been removed, the vagina is closed at the top and the abdomen stitched or clamped closed. As you wake up, you may find you are feeling sick, and that your abdomen is hurting. You will find that you have a drip attached to your arm for liquid or blood, and a catheter to drain off fluids from your bladder. You will also have a drain in your pelvis and possibly one from the wound.

The recovery from hysterectomy varies from woman to woman. There is no single universal reaction, but you can expect to experience some discomfort. At first you will only be allowed sips of fluid, to make sure your system can cope as it gets back to normal.

The wound drain will probably be removed within a day, and the pelvic drain in about a week. The catheter will go when you are able to cope without it – from a day or two to several days. You will be encouraged to move around to prevent blood clots.

If you have had your ovaries removed you may start to experience hot flushes, as the menopause starts. You may be offered hormone replacement therapy (HRT), to offset these symptoms. If for some reason your consultant says it would be unwise for you to have HRT, then ask him/her to explain why, and check whether instead you could have one of the other substitutes that can relieve the symptoms.

The after-effects of hysterectomy can last a while. You may have a reduced bladder capacity, and have to retrain your bladder. You may find you need to make love carefully until your newly shortened vagina gets stretched again.

You may also feel weepy and need lots of reassurance from your partner. He/she will also be coping with their own emotional reaction; many of the women I talked to found that going through this thing together actually brought them closer to their partners. Try to get lots of cuddles and physical affection if you can, and give

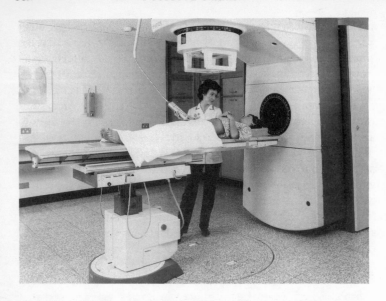

Figure 9. Having external radiotherapy at the Cromwell Hospital.

yourself and your partner time and space to discuss how you feel about what has happened.

Radiotherapy

In radiotherapy high-energy rays destroy the cancer. It can be used in a number of ways: before a hysterectomy to shrink the tumour; after a hysterectomy to destroy the last remnant of cancer cells, or 'knock it on the head' as Jane B. said; or often on its own instead of surgery. It can be used internally and externally.

The first step is to plan your treatment, and for this you'll go to the radiotherapy department for a few exploratory visits. The radiographer will do a Pelvic CT or CAT scan to find out just where the radium treatment is needed. As described on page 62 a tampon will first be placed in your vagina and a liquid put into your anus. Remember that the nurses are used to doing this, and that a little embarrassment is worth it when it is saving your life.

You usually have external radiotherapy as an out-patient and will probably have to attend hospital three or four times a week, over perhaps six weeks. The radiographer will make marks on your skin, and then position you on a couch under the machine. The treatment may take several minutes, but it usually isn't painful, 'just boring' as one woman said. You will usually be able to communicate with the nurses through an intercom, and they will be watching you on a closed circuit television to check that you are all right.

Internal radiotherapy is usually done in hospital and you will be in a room on your own; plastic applicators are placed inside your vagina and inside these are put radioactive caesium rods. You have to lie very still so that they don't move and only affect the area they are meant to heal. You should feel little pain, though taking the applicators out can be painful, and of course lying still for ages is uncomfortable. 'I got very lonely' said one woman I talked to, as she described how visitors and nurses could not come in so that they would not be affected by the radiation.

Both of these treatments can have side effects: Sue said that she was 'very near giving up at one point; it didn't seem worth it.' Nausea, diarrhoea and a cystitis-like pain when passing water can occur and make your life very uncomfortable, and you will feel tired and weepy a lot of the time. But many hospitals give tablets to cope with all these side effects, and they do not last for ever.

Even if you haven't had a hysterectomy, radiotherapy will stop your ovaries working and you will experience menopausal symptoms. Again, ask for hormone replacement therapy if you want to. Just as with hysterectomy, you may feel depressed at the thought of not being able to have children – allow yourself all the support you need, and give yourself time to recover.

Chemotherapy

In chemotherapy drugs are used to destroy cancer cells. It is usually administered when the cancer has spread to various parts of your body, and is not often used for cervical cancer; its use will depend on your particular illness.

The drugs damage the cells to stop them dividing and are given over a period of time which can vary from a few weeks to several months. They are usually injected into a vein, though sometimes they may be swallowed as tablets or capsules.

They affect normal cells as well as cancer cells, and therefore have a number of side effects. You can get very tired and will need to rest a lot. You will vomit, and may have ulcers on your mouth. You won't however, with the usual form of chemotherapy used for cervical cancer, lose your hair.

As your blood cells are affected, you are vulnerable to infections, so you need to build up your general health as much as you can. If you do catch an infection, the hospital will usually treat it with antibiotics or even blood transfusions.

Final thoughts

All these radical treatments can sound horrendous but don't let things get out of proportion. If you are reading this book having just been diagnosed CIN 1 or 2, then most of this information is probably not relevant to you at all. Read about it to find out what can happen to other women, but don't panic.

If you have CIN 3, then similarly you have an excellent chance of only ever experiencing these treatments by reading about them since they are usually only used if you have invasive cancer.

If you do have to have one or more of these treatments, that is tough to handle. You will need support and you will need to be flexible and brave. But if the women I have talked to are anything to go by, you will make some meaning out of what is happening, and you will be able to look back in a few years and see it all in a new perspective. And perhaps tell other women who are going through it how you survived . . .

7

PREVENTION

> Now, I feel I'm doing something to take charge . . . I'm
> taking control of my own health. (Tracey)

What do you need to do in order never to have a positive smear? Or
in the case of those of us who have had one, whether we needed
treatment or not, what can we do in order never to have one again?

The first step, I think, is to realize that we have a choice. There
are things we can do that make us vulnerable, and there are things
we can do to make us less vulnerable. We are adults now, and no
one is going to shout at us if we do some of the 'wrong' things and
miss out some of the 'right' things. Admittedly some of the
Government warnings and some of the quoted medical professionals speak to us like children, telling us that if we aren't good
little girls, the bogyman will come and get us. Some of them also
tell us that it is our fault that the bogyman is on the loose at all.

We do still have a choice. If we choose, we can avoid positive
smears, we can go some way to avoiding cervical cancer altogether
by following all the guidelines for its prevention. Or if we choose
we can adopt some of them, and leave the rest to fate. If instead we
smoke heavily, are on the Pill, make love unprotected with a new
man every night, we are in effect stacking the odds against
ourselves, and that is our choice.

Prevention possibilities

Build your health

Almost anything you do to build your health will give you a better
chance of not developing cervical conditions. Many infections,

which are breeding grounds for CIN, develop when we are run down. CIN and cancer can advance more rapidly if our immune systems are low and not working properly. A body that is fighting the debilitating effects of being overweight, of foods that stimulate allergies, or under-exercised heart and lungs, will be less able to cope with fighting off illness than a body that is running like a well-tuned engine.

The following are some guidelines and things to think about when deciding how to build your health and strengthen your immune system.

Food. A good diet is essential to health. 'We cut out fat and sugar, and we eat salads, fish and chicken.' (Sue). Eating unrefined foods such as whole grains will give you a healthier, high-fibre diet. Fresh fruit and vegetables contain more vitamins than canned or frozen.

Avoid any foods that you feel you are allergic to. Common allergies are to coffee, tea, wheat and dairy products, so if you suspect you have a bad reaction to any of these, try cutting them out of your diet and re-introducing them one at a time. Foods that contain flavourings and colourings, or have been sprayed with pesticide can affect you too, so check pre-packed foods for E numbers and avoid them if you can.

Don't diet constantly. In fact, try not to diet at all; denying your body essential nutrients can do more harm than good. Instead, try to eat a balanced diet and burn off the excess calories through exercise. If you have an eating problem, such as anorexia nervosa or bulimia, or even suspect that you have, ask your GP to refer you for expert help immediately.

Drugs. Limit your alcohol intake. Try not to drink more than two or three standard drinks two or three times a week. Keep clear of all kinds of hard drug, and if you can, avoid using soft drugs, pain-killers or tranquillizers. Obviously if you have been prescribed them by your doctor you should first check with her/him that this will be all right.

Vitamins. Find good prolonged-release nutrition multi-vitamin and mineral tablets to take each day. Make sure you take enough vitamin C (particularly if you smoke), B vitamins (particularly if you are on the Pill), and vitamin A.

Exercise. Take regular exercise. The best is a combination of regular and vigorous exercise during each week. This could include some regular gentle exercise to build stamina, and two or three bouts of vigorous exercise to get your heart and lungs working. A regular walk to work, an exercise class and a swimming session would be ideal. Don't try to exercise if you hate it – but find some sort of exercise (dance, competitive games, running) that you can get enthusiastic about. If you get bored exercising, buy a personal stereo – or find a companion.

Relaxation. Take some time every day to relax and allow yourself to assimilate what you have done and seen. Meditation, stress reduction, yoga, relaxation tapes or simply sitting and thinking will do.

Check-ups. Have a regular yearly check-up that includes a check on blood pressure, heart, kidneys, ovaries. Your local FPA should be able to tell you how to check your own breasts monthly for lumps.

Stop smoking

In my parents' day, smoking was the fashionable thing to do. Nowadays, it is becoming distinctly unfashionable. Very few of the women I spoke to smoked. One gave up immediately after her hysterectomy. Only a few chain-smoked their way through the interview.

Stopping smoking will decrease your risk of getting cervical cancer – that is a fact. It will also increase your ability to run, play, work, make love – and breathe. Your skin will look better and you will be less likely to die of heart and lung disease. But if you do smoke, none of this may matter. Even the thought of cervical cancer can seem a long way away while the thought of the next cigarette is all-attractive. There are ways to stop smoking, although to date no one has discovered one which always works for everyone. You could try one of the patent remedies available in chemists' shops. You could read one of a number of 'stop smoking' books. You could simply look at what you get out of smoking – relaxation, social acceptance, a sense of elegance – and try getting these things elsewhere. Many counsellors offer stop-smoking cures; the most successful are often based on hypnotherapy, in which your sub-conscious mind is invited to help you find other things to do rather than smoke.

It could be that one of these methods works for you. Perhaps, like one of the women I spoke to, you are able to 'stop just like that' once you realize that to continue could lead to another positive smear.

Cleanliness

Keeping clean is one obvious way to minimize the risk of develop-ing cervical cancer. Washing genitals, particularly before making love, is both sensible and can be extremely erotic if you do it together. And if you or your partner live or work in a 'dirty' area, where chemicals, diesel fuel, asbestos or mining dirt is in the air, then it is absolutely essential. Some sources also say that neither of you should use talcum powder on your genitals, and that perfumed tampons should also be avoided.

In a more general sense, fight for better working and living conditions – showers at work, bathrooms and washing machines in the home – both for yourself and other women at risk.

Coming off the Pill

As I explain in the chapter on Causes, there is some evidence to suggest that taking the contraceptive pill increases the likelihood of abnormal cervical conditions. Changing to another method of contraception will reduce this risk. The main options are: natural birth control, IUCD, barrier methods such as the cap or the condom.

Natural birth control needs a lot of knowledge and dedication to make it work, but its advantages are that it doesn't involve the insertion of a foreign body in your cervix, as the IUCD does, or chemicals in your vagina, as some barrier methods do. However, it

CONDOM . . . . IN POSITION
Can be bought over the counter
and from vending machines

'DUTCH'
CAP

CERVICAL
CAP

The right size has to be prescribed
before purchase

Figure 10a. Barrier contraception methods. You will notice that only the condom gives complete protection against the transmission of viruses.

APPLICATOR screwed onto a tube of
CONTRACEPTIVE JELLY
— ready for filling

SPERMICIDAL
PESSARY

Figure 10b. These are often used in conjunction with barrier contraception methods.

is notoriously unreliable (18–24 per cent failure rate) and demands a great deal of self- (and partner-) control.

The IUCD allows for spontaneity, but is not 100 per cent fail-safe and does make you vulnerable to infection (I speak as one who knows . . .). If you have just had treatment for a positive smear, you will know that you need to have the IUCD removed during treatment, and may have to wait a while for it to be re-inserted.

Barrier methods are less spontaneous than the Pill, but have the advantage of protecting you from possible infections. If you are in a stable relationship and are taking the Pill, but would like to change to a barrier method, it might be a good idea to discuss this first with your partner. He may feel that this will spoil the spontaneity of making love or he may be worried about the increased possibility of your becoming pregnant. If you want him to wear a condom he may feel threatened or that he is being asked to take too much responsibility.

If you are not in a regular relationship, then you will have to learn how to explain to a new partner that you are using a method of contraception that involves some forethought.

Barrier methods of contraception

At the time of going to press, the evidence linking sexual experience and cervical cancer is unclear. In particular, as mentioned in the section of this book on Causes, there is conflicting evidence of the link between the wart virus and cervical conditions.

Many women are choosing to use barrier contraception, to protect themselves against a possible 'cancer trigger' from their partner. This is true even when a woman has only one partner, and has been with him for many years: 'I won't have sex without a condom now, and I'm sure throughout my life I'll always use one.' (Julie). It is unclear from the evidence whether these women are being extremely wise or far too panicky. Current media publicity suggests the former. Several doctors I spoke to also said that women were wise to protect themselves. 'In the United States, they recommend all positive smear patients to use barrier contraception for life,' said one consultant. Also, a study in treating CIN conditions by using barrier methods showed remarkable effectiveness (see page 40).

Conversely, some doctors believe, and have told patients, that there is only a coincidental link between making love unprotected and developing cervical conditions, and that there are so many other possible things that could trigger CIN that using barrier contraception may be irrelevant. Few doctors suggested to women I interviewed that they should use barrier methods of contraception as a way of preventing further development of CIN.

At the same time many doctors indicated that once a woman has received treatment for CIN, any viruses may well be effectively removed. 'There was evidence of the wart virus,' Anna was told, 'but it will have gone now.' Although we know that the virus can remain in the folds of the vagina, these doctors were confident enough of the unlikelihood of its precipitating cervical abnormality and so did not suggest using barrier contraception. In addition, recent research mentioned in the chapter on Causes (see page 104), showed that follow-up studies of women who had had the wart virus HPV-16 and had received laser treatment for CIN showed little recurrence of abnormal cells. Another study has shown no evidence of partners reinfecting each other with the wart virus after treatment for CIN.

Between the 'always use barrier contraception' lobby, and the 'it's not relevant' lobby, I found it difficult to come to a firm conclusion. The nearest to common sense I seemed to get is this: you obviously want to protect yourself from all infections and viruses, whether or not they are relevant to cervical cancer, so you will probably choose barrier methods of contraception, unless you and your partner show no evidence of any virus, and you both only sleep with each other. (There may be a factor other than the wart virus – for example, your partner's sperm – which is responsible for cervical cancer, but you might want to take that risk!)

Remember too that viruses are not only present when symptoms show – they can develop or remain, and you will have to take a decision whether to chance this or not. Even if you have never had a virus, you could have contracted one from your last sexual partner. You can certainly check – if your partner is willing and doesn't mind the discomfort – that he is not infected with the wart virus, by asking him to dab a mild vinegar and water solution over his penis. Infected areas will show up white when examined with a magnifying glass. This won't, of course, give you information about whether you yourself are clear of the virus.

If you are not clear of herpes or wart virus, or your partner is not clear or will not go to be checked, then you can protect yourself by using a barrier method. If you have no regular partner, you could use a barrier method until you are sure that each partner is not carrying any virus. Asking a new partner to go for a check-up can be embarrassing, but once you are sure you have a steady relationship, it may be worthwhile.

A last, intriguing thought: Mary reports going on a course for safer sex which included the erotic possibilities of inserting caps and putting on condoms. A lovely idea – could your evening institute run a course like that . . . ?

Not making love

Two of the women I spoke to had done this. Hilda said: 'If sex was going to cause that many problems, I decided I wouldn't have any more relationships . . . until I'd done what I wanted to in my career.'

This might be a real possibility for you, particularly if as a result of your positive smear experience you are feeling bitter about your partner, or about men in general. Remember though that abnormal cervical conditions may result from a number of factors, and not making love that involves penetration does not mean that your safety is guaranteed.

It is also significant that some media coverage of the cervical cancer problem hints that until women stop making love then they will continue to get cervical cancer. I hope no woman will fall for this victim-blame by ceasing to make love out of guilt.

Screening

Interestingly, when newspaper headlines or medical journals talk about prevention, they usually mean screening – in other words, the smear test.

It seems strange to me to call it prevention when what is happening is merely diagnosis – a bit like a dentist suggesting that you come for regular check-ups but don't bother to clean your teeth. The argument is that if we call screening prevention, then women will feel they are involved and are taking charge – and this is a good point. But I would prefer to see women taking charge at a much earlier stage in the process. Much of the screening would be rendered unnecessary if we took care of the primary prevention.

One doctor at present is indeed recommending that screening be stopped.[3] He points out that the rates of cervical cancer in some countries have not gone down appreciably since screening was introduced, and that some studies have shown that cervical cancer is found as much in women who have been screened as in those who haven't. His opponents argue that the rates have not dropped because other factors, such as the wart virus, have increased the cancer rates just as the screening procedures were decreasing it.

What does this mean for you? While screening does not alter the statistics, and certainly does not prevent, only diagnose, it is certainly worth using it as a tool in your own health care. *Remember that the occurrence of invasive cancer in women who are regularly screened is practically zero*. 'Go to the Family Planning Clinic and lie if you have to in order to get a regular smear,' said Sue. 'Once every five years is ridiculous.' As somebody who did lie and so got a smear test after one year instead of five – therefore surviving CIN 3 – I have to admit that what she says rings true.

Up to now, few clinics or doctors have 'reminded' women that it is time for them to have a smear test, so you need to take responsibility for your own screening process. Happily however, there is now more awareness of the need for a computerized recall system; some health authorities are now aiming at a recall for every woman between the ages of 20 and 64 every three years, and this is certainly a step forward. You can sometimes get smear tests through your local GP, certainly through your local Family Planning Clinic and Well Woman Clinics. If you have any problem finding facilities, ring your local Community Health Council.

On the other hand, I wonder if having such screening is covering up, for the authorities and for women, the need for real prevention. Why not inform women of what they can do to help themselves rather than allow them to live in ignorance and then harangue them to go for screening and be grateful that 'the system' spots what is wrong.

What now?

We don't really know what causes cervical cancer, and until we do there can be no foolproof prevention. In the meantime, there are ways we can make ourselves less vulnerable. There are ways we can decrease the odds.

A final very positive thought is that if you have had an abnormal smear, and through treatment have had your condition cured, then you are in the lowest possible risk bracket in the future. Once you have then had a clear result, you have a much lower than average chance of getting the condition again. You are in fact in a better position than women who have never had a positive smear.

And if having a positive smear is the mechanism by which we stop and think about our health, and choose a healthier life style, then in fact for some women, it is worth it. 'Before, I used to feel ill a lot,' said Anna. 'Now, things are going really well.'

8

WHAT ARE THE FACTS?

I was sure the more I knew and understood, the better I'd
be. (Linda)

Knowledge is power. Knowing what is happening to you makes
you far less vulnerable, and means that you can cope with what is
going on. Understanding the facts and knowing what you are
talking about when speaking to a doctor means that you can
address her/him with authority.

There is a danger. If you know some things and not others, you
can get frightened. Janet 'panicked at a section in a book about
lymph involvement in cancer patients – and I'd only just got my
smear test result . . .' So if you want the facts, get them in a
balanced way, not in a way that makes you panic.

Where to get information

There are very few books and leaflets on the market, so this is
definitely an opportunity to develop your initiative. You will need
to have a great deal of persistence too – and a large dictionary to
help with the medical terms, but there are ways of getting general
and specific information.

First, ask your own doctor, and when the time comes, the
consultant. They are experts on the disease, even though they are
not always expert at explaining things. Remember that a book will
give you generalities – only your own doctor can discuss your
particular case with you. Elsewhere in this book we suggest specific
questions you might want to ask. Some medical professionals don't
realize that women need to know what is happening and many

women spoke of having to ask their doctors repeatedly for general information about cervical conditions, and specific information about their condition in particular. 'Tell women to sit there until they get the information,' recommended Julia – and this is exactly what many women had to do.

The hospital you go to will very likely have its own information leaflets setting out the relevant facts in simple language. These are often written by staff or ex-patients who have been through it all themselves. They rarely address emotional issues; their strength is the clear presentation of facts. But you may need to ask for them, as they are often not readily available. If your hospital hasn't got a leaflet, suggest they get some copies of the excellent ones published by the Women's Health and Reproductive Rights Information Centre (address in Resource Section of this book) – or even offer to write them yourself! Diana did: 'I ended up preparing the leaflets for them.'

While waiting to see the doctor and the specialist though, you can gain a lot of useful background knowledge. Many of the women I spoke to got up at some point during our conversation and said 'I'll just go and get the file . . .' The idea of The File, into which you put all the information you are gathering, became a catch phrase. So start your own 'File'!

Try reading some of the leaflets and books mentioned in the Resource section at the back of this book. Getting books out from the library is also often worthwhile as the coverage of cervical conditions in many general health books is so small that often it's not worth buying them. If you feel uncomfortable about borrowing such books from the library, you are not alone: 'I hid them under a general health book and smuggled them out,' said Linda.

There are also some videos that you can buy, and though they are not cheap, maybe your local FPC could be persuaded to pay the cost if you ran a women's evening to show them. The better alternative is usually to hire. See the Resource section for details.

You can also keep an eye open in newspapers, magazines and on the television and radio for news of recent developments on the cervical cancer front. 'Once you know about it, you pick up little snippets from everywhere,' (Rosemary). But be prepared for biased reporting. It isn't news to say: 'Most women need minor treatment after a positive smear.' It is news to dwell on the once-a-decade horror story.

A final way to gain knowledge is to talk to other women. But remember that many of them, like you, will be scared and upset, and their stories will reflect this and stress the unhappy bits. That said, women supporting women by passing on accounts of their own condition is probably one of the best kinds of information you will get. It is, after all, based on first-hand experience.

In this book, I am aiming only to give the basics. As one woman said: 'Simple, everyday language please; I'm not in the mood for long words.' If you want more detailed information, a more medically-based guide to cervical cancer will help you.

The basics

Your reproductive system

Your womb is nestled inside your pelvis for comfort and protection. On either side of it lie the ovaries which hold the eggs. The base of the womb, situated at the top of the vagina, is called the

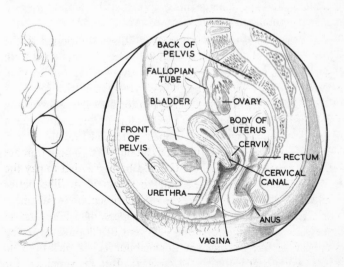

Figure 11. Your reproductive system.

cervix. After love-making, your partner's sperm travels from the vagina through a small opening in the cervix, up the cervical canal, and into the womb. Every month during your period, the lining of the womb detaches itself and flows down the cervical canal, through the cervix and into the vagina.

Various other organs are situated around the womb. Most, like the kidneys and bladder, are responsible for getting rid of waste products from your body. Some, like the lymph glands, protect your body against disease.

The cervix is fairly well protected by being inside your body, but since it comes into contact with the outside environment it is also quite vulnerable.

Finding out about the cervix

It's still quite rare for a woman to feel comfortable about exploring the sexual parts of her body. We don't have the advantages that men do, with 'everything on the outside'!

But we do have a natural tendency to touch parts of our bodies that are not well – as you will know when you have a mouth ulcer or bitten cheek, and your tongue inexorably drifts back to it time and again. So it is totally natural to want to begin to come to terms with your cervix by exploring it and finding out more about it.

If you want to, stand with one foot on a chair, or lie flat on your back with your knees up. Put your finger carefully inside your vagina. (Wash your hands first, and make sure your nails are short in case you scratch yourself.) Feel inside your vagina to the end; the cervix is there. Some women describe it as a 'dome shape', a 'lump', a 'bump with a dip in it'. It feels firmer than the soft walls of the vagina, and as one woman said: 'Once you've found it, you'll know . . .'

Those of us who use the cap, which involves checking that the cervix is covered each time we put it in, will be used to this. The rest of us may take some time to find out which is cervix and which is the rest of our vagina. Remember too that the cervix alters position according to the time of the month and how aroused you are – so don't worry if you 'lose' it occasionally.

If you want you can also buy a speculum, an instrument which

Figure 12. Exploring your vagina and cervix.

allows you to hold your vagina open and explore it more fully. The Women's Health and Reproductive Rights Information Centre (details in the Resource section) sell a speculum kit that you can use. The speculum is shaped like two shoehorns joined together. When you place it inside the opening to your vagina (warm it first!) the two halves can be eased apart, allowing you to explore your vagina more fully. It is a good idea to use a mirror so that you can see into your vagina, as well as feel inside it.

Whether you are looking or just touching, try to notice as many things as you can. Be aware of moisture or discharge, and of the shape, size and feel of your cervix. Become familiar with these things. Remember that this part of your body is undergoing changes, so it may feel particularly vulnerable at the moment.

Figure 13. The transformation zone of the cervix.

The cervix – types of skin

Inside the cervix, beyond the reach of your fingers, the cells of the skin are soft and have a good blood supply. They are called columnar cells. At the outside of the cervix, and in the vagina, the cells are of a different kind: they are called squamous cells and have less of a blood supply than columnar cells, and are 'harder', so that you don't bleed every time you are penetrated when making love.

Between the two types of skin is a transformation zone, where cells change from one kind to another. The soft, columnar cells inside the cervical canal change into harder squamous cells towards the outside of the cervix. This is a way of protecting the vulnerable cervix from the outside world. The medical term for this transition is squamous metaplasia.

You won't be able to feel the different kinds of cell, or feel the change from one kind to another. If you have an internal examination to check your cervix after a positive smear, the consultant may use a high-powered microscope to see the different kinds of cell – and sometimes, if you are interested, she can show you photos of your own cervical cells.

What can go wrong

Infections. One thing that can go wrong in your cervix, or vagina, is that you may catch an infection of some sort. Thrush is a common infection which causes irritation and a discharge. Another common infection is trichomoniasis, which also results in a vaginal discharge. Nowadays almost all such infections are completely treatable, but they can cause your smear result to be unclear. If you do have an infection, the doctor will often suggest you have a repeat smear after treatment.

Viruses. Your cervix and vagina may also be attacked by a virus. In particular the viruses that carry herpes and warts are relevant to your having a positive smear. Both viruses are infectious and can be passed on through skin contact.

The herpes virus is caught through skin to skin contact, although some people are immune to it. It can lie dormant, but can also flare up when a person is stressed, to cause red spots which turn to painful, weeping blisters.

Warts are growths that can occur on many parts of the body. They are caused by a virus called human papilloma virus, of which there are several kinds. Certain kinds create genital warts, found on the penis in men and the vagina, cervix and external sexual parts in women. However it often exists in the body without producing warts at all, so it is very difficult to track down. A simple test for penile warts is to swab a mild solution of vinegar and water over the penis – infected areas then show up as small white patches.

Cervical erosion. Usually, the cells on the surface of the cervix are the hard, squamous cells, and the ones on the inside are the softer, columnar cells. If the softer cells come to the surface of the cervix, this can be a problem. Because they are softer, they are more vulnerable. They can become inflamed, cause a discharge or bleed easily if touched.

This is called 'cervical erosion' or 'ectopy'. It sounds as if the cervix is being rubbed or 'eroded' away, but this is an exaggeration. Cervical erosion can happen during ovulation, menstruation, in pregnancy, or when a girl starts having her periods, and it can also be caused by the Pill. Many women get it, and unless you have an abnormal smear, it's usually agreed to be harmless.

Abnormally developing cells. The cells on the cervix can develop in abnormal ways. The cells in the transformation zone are particularly vulnerable to abnormal change and may begin to change towards becoming cancer cells. It is important to realize that this is not a change to cancer, but a change in that direction. It happens gradually and slowly, and there are various stages before the cells become truly cancerous. It can take between ten and twenty years for cells to become cancerous. This is why, of all the cancers we know, cervical cancer is one of the easiest to spot and to stop in good time.

One medical term for such changes in the surface layers of the cervix is dysplasia. Another term is pre-cancer, and this can be misleading, because you can start to think that you are definitely going to develop true cancer. In fact, some abnormally changing cells never develop into cancer, even if they are not treated. A third term to describe abnormal cell changes is cervical intraepithelial neoplasia. If you find this a mouthful, you are not alone! It is such a mouthful that it is usually shortened to CIN. Throughout this book I have preferred to use this expression when discussing early, pre-cancerous changes.

In order to make distinctions between various stages of change, doctors have developed a scale, according to how much of the cervix is affected:

CIN 1 means that only the top third of the cells on the surface of the cervix are affected.

CIN 2 means that two thirds of the cells are affected.

CIN 3 means that all the cells on the surface are affected.

Another way of describing CIN 3 is carcinoma in situ. The word carcinoma means cancer, and if you see this term on your medical sheet, or overhear it, as Anna did ('I heard the consultant say those words on his way into the room to examine me . . .') you may well, as she did, panic. There is no need to. Carcinoma in situ is not yet true cancer, as explained later in this chapter.

To get things in perspective, remember that even if left untreated, many cases of CIN 1 and 2 can go back to normal. It has even been known for cases of CIN 3 to change back. And remember too that most women who have treatment for these pre-cancerous conditions never develop cancer.

Cancer. Beyond the CIN scale are further scales of seriousness. The cells of the cervix may indeed be cancerous.

How does cancer happen? Healthy cells grow regularly by dividing and making more cells. This is how children grow. When this division stops, growth stops – and this is why older people change in their appearance, as cells stop reproducing, and wrinkles begin.

When cells grow at an abnormal rate, and the growth gets out of control, this is called a tumour. It can be harmless (benign) or harmful (malignant). Malignant cells are those which spread far beyond their starting point, and destroy other parts of the body, affecting other areas by creating new tumours called 'secondaries'.

Cervical cancer is almost always caused by abnormal changes in the squamous and columnar cells, as described on page 84. This abnormal change spreads beyond the surface layer of the skin and invades the cervix. There is another form of cervical cancer called adenocarcinoma which doesn't begin in the transformation zone, but in the tissues of the canal that runs through the cervix. As far as we know it is not caused by the same factors as the cervical cancer discussed in this book, and it is extremely rare indeed.

If left untreated cancer spreads further into the cervix. It can invade the whole of the pelvis, and then attack the lymph nodes and bloodstream.

There are several grades of cancer, just as there are several grades of CIN. Only the very last grades are fatal. 54 per cent of all women with diagnosed cervical cancer survive it, and 95 per cent of those with the earliest grades survive. The highest mortality rates are

SURFACE CELLS

BASE MEMBRANE

UNDERLYING TISSUE OF CERVIX

NORMAL   CIN   INVASIVE CARCINOMA

CERVIX   VAGINA

Stage I
The tumour is confined
to the cervix

WALL OF PELVIS   LYMPH NODES

Stage II
The tumour has spread to
the vagina and neighbouring tissue

Stage III
The tumour extends
to the pelvic wall

Stage IV
The tumour extends
beyond the pelvis

Figure 14. Stages of CIN.

found in those women who, unlike you, have never had a smear test.

When is it pre-cancer and when is it cancer?

This is one of the main mixed messages in the whole of the 'positive smear' area. It is confusing because, in the majority of cases, we are dealing with a condition that develops along a continuum. Mild cases are nowhere near being cancerous, more severe cases are more likely to be so.

The dividing line that doctors draw relates to what cancer does: it spreads and grows. This is the very nature of cancer, to grow and invade the body it attacks. So if the condition is not invading the cells at a deep level, it is not regarded as truly cancerous. The words and terminology doctors use refer to whether the condition has started to spread beyond the very surface cells of the cervix. If the condition is only affecting surface cells, it is easily treated and there will be no danger of its having invaded the body. This is the condition that doctors call CIN. It is not seen as cancer yet because it has not yet started to invade. The grades of CIN, as we have seen, refer to the extent to which the cervix is affected by this surface condition – a third (mild), two thirds (moderate) or all (severe). The final grade, CIN 3 is, confusingly, called by the same Latin name as is used for true cancer – *carcinoma* – but if the condition has not yet invaded, it is not seen as true cancer.

If the condition has spread beyond the surface cells of the cervix, then doctors consider it has invaded: they use the term 'invasive carcinoma', and see the condition as cancer. The treatment has to be more searching in order to eradicate all of the affected cells.

A positive smear test only reveals whether the cells are abnormal or not; the term used is whether they are dyskaryotic. If the dyskaryosis is mild, it is very unlikely that the abnormality has spread so far that it is invasive. If it is moderate or severe, there is usually little chance. But a smear test doesn't test for CIN or cancer; you need a biopsy for this.

So if your smear shows mild dyskaryosis, it is practically certain that the condition you have is not invasive and therefore not true cancer. You may have an examination or biopsy to make sure, but minimal treatment will be needed. And as the condition can develop, some doctors will refer you for an examination as a matter of course – particularly as with today's waiting lists, if you need to enter the treatment cycle at all, you need to get in early.

With moderate or severe dyskaryosis, a doctor will usually consider what other symptoms you have if any. S/he will send you to hospital for an examination and a biopsy to make sure that you are not one of the few women who have an invasive condition.

If, when the examinations have been done, you are told you have a CIN condition, you know that the abnormal cells are only on the surface of the skin. Various proportions of your cervix could be affected depending on whether you have CIN 1, 2, or 3, but the

Figure 15. Preparing for a smear test.

condition has not invaded, and is therefore not regarded as cancer. If however it has gone below the surface of the skin, then you are no longer seen as having a CIN condition, but true 'invasive carcinoma'.

The two are on a continuum though, and this is why there may sometimes be confusion. If you have CIN you will be advised to go for treatment because, left alone, it might spread and become invasive cancer – but doctors will still reassure you by saying that it 'isn't yet'. In the same way, advertising campaigns for the smear test talk of cervical cancer, even though the majority of the positive results show CIN conditions, not invasive conditions.

As I mentioned before, the length of time it takes for CIN to turn to cancer, if in fact it does, can be anything up to twenty years – although there seems to be a new, fast developing form of the condition which can become serious in a much shorter time.

If you can become clear in your mind about the relationship between the two things, you will be well on your way to avoiding the trap of mixed messages.

What is a smear test?

The smear test we use nowadays was developed in the 1940s by an Italian physician called Papanicolau. The smear is sometimes called a Pap smear, after him. Its strength is that it picks up early signs of cervical problems, before true cancer takes a hold.

(a)
with a spatula

(b)
with a swab-stick
in the cervical canal

Figure 16. Taking a smear test.

If, as is likely, you have had a smear test before reading this book, then you will know what it involves. The doctor will ask you to lie down on the couch and will open your vagina with a speculum. S/he will scrape a spatula around your cervix in a complete circle, trying to make sure that s/he has gathered a sample of all the cells around the neck of the womb.

The doctor will then spread the cells on to a glass slide. The slide is stained so that individual cells can be easily seen. It is then taken to a laboratory to be examined under a microscope by a specially trained technician. The smear can show a number of things: it might show such things as whether you have a coil or IUCD fitted; it can show up inflammation or infection; it can tell you whether you have a virus such as the herpes or wart virus. And a cervical smear can also tell you about the dyskaryosis just mentioned. It cannot however tell you whether severely changing cells are yet invasive, so the doctors need to do further tests to be sure of this.

Because a smear test can provide all this information, one condition of the cervix may sometimes hide another. If you have an infection, for example, the smear may be difficult to read and the laboratory technician will be unable to tell whether the cells show

Figure 17. Your smear test result form.

abnormal changes or not. In this case, the doctor will often be asked to do the test again. And if so, it's usually wise to clear up any such problems before re-doing the smear.

After the smear test has been examined, the results are noted on a standard form and returned to your doctor. This is the point at which, if the results are positive, you will get the news.

While this book was in preparation, a new method of screening was developed. It involves using a camera to take pictures of the cervix and so check for abnormalities. If it proves effective, this may well make screening easier and more accurate, thus encouraging more women to go for regular check-ups.

What now?

You have now had the benefit of a short guided tour around the facts of a 'positive smear'. It may take some time for you to be able to understand and assimilate these facts. One woman spoke of not being able to 'take anything in until it was all over'. Also, many of these facts are not relevant to you, and you will never need to know them.

Whatever your positive smear means, it is an opportunity to get to know more about your body.

9

WHAT ARE THE CAUSES?

I didn't search for reasons or causes because I wasn't looking for things to blame. (Julie)

Why is it happening? This is a question that every woman I talked to wondered about. They wondered in a general way and in a specific way, about what caused cervical cancer and CIN. They asked: why is it happening to me?

This question can be a cry to heaven – or whatever your substitute for heaven is. It can be a question that doesn't expect an answer; you simply feel angry and resentful that such a thing can be happening. You have every right to be angry and resentful, for what is happening to you is not pleasant. And if you want to, you can channel your anger into an energy for doing something practical – exploring what laid the foundations for your condition, and what can stop it happening again.

Finding out why

If you do decide to explore these things, you will need all the energy you can get. Because of all the questions surrounding the issue of positive smear, the actual 'cause' of cervical cancer is one of the most difficult.

Doctors disagree, medical professionals argue, the press claims one thing, pressure groups claim another. The women I spoke to came up with several possible links which the professionals had never even considered. If you are looking for clear-cut answers, you won't get them.

You should also be aware that you are touching upon an area in which people may react strongly and negatively. If you decide to explore the issue, you are likely to come across opinions that will upset you, make you angry, put you on the defensive. For people are very ready to blame, dramatize, blandly reassure or simply refuse to comment. As Frances said: 'No one told me why it happened – and I hated that.'

We still don't know for sure what the causes of cervical cancers are: it will take many more years of research, argument and unhappiness before we reach anything approaching a satisfactory answer. All I can offer in this chapter is a path through the minefield, a guide to recent thoughts on the subject.

Causes or vulnerabilities?

Let us start by challenging the idea of a 'cause' of cervical cancer and CIN. We are not talking about an injury, such as a broken leg, that is caused by an accident.

We don't yet know what makes a cell decide to grow and go on growing out of control. It is not yet clear what the trigger is. But although we do not know what 'causes' cancer, we do know that certain conditions make the cells more vulnerable to cancer taking hold. So when we talk of causes, we are talking in fact about factors that create vulnerability.

It is important to remember this. Many newspaper articles, television programmes and top medical consultants forget it. Every factor mentioned here as being present in women who develop cervical CIN or cancer, may also be present in women who don't develop it. So if any of them are present in your life, then that doesn't mean to say you will get cancer. It just means that you are more vulnerable. And the more of these factors you have in your life, the more vulnerable you are. In the same way as if you go jumping off cliffs you are more likely to get injured than if you stay at home reading. You are not under a death sentence – but you are stacking the odds against yourself.

Vulnerability factors

Diet

The links made between diet and cervical pre-cancers and cancers
are still uncertain. However, vulnerability is a wide-ranging thing.
If your diet is unhealthy or unbalanced; if it makes you severely
over or underweight for your size, it's making you vulnerable
anyway. Many of the women I spoke to had improved their diet
after having a positive smear.

Some foods can lower the efficiency of your immune system
which helps you fight disease. Generally, foods which have an
adverse effect on any part of your body (such as too much fat,
caffeine or alcohol) increase your vulnerability to disease of any
kind.

Recent American work has suggested that women with cervical
pre-cancers or cancers often have deficiencies of certain elements –
vitamin C, beta carotene and folic acid. So a diet deficient in any of
these is unwise.

Vitamin C helps to convert harmful substances in the bloodstream into non-harmful ones, and is found in uncooked fruit and
vegetables. Beta carotene, found in carrots and other yellow
vegetables and fruits, helps to build up resistance to disease. The
contraceptive pill makes it difficult to absorb the folic acid from
what you eat, so you are particularly liable to deficiency if you are
on the Pill.

The environment

It has been recognized for a long time that a dirty environment and
disease go together. Recent studies have shown a link between
'dirty' jobs and a higher incidence of positive smears in women
workers or the wives of male workers.[4] Workers (or their wives) in
the forces, the mines, at furnaces and foundries, on farms and on
fishing boats, in mills, have all been found to be more at risk.

Think of the proven risks of asbestos, which now has been
removed from work places and schools. It's easy to see why if you
work with such high-risk substances you are more vulnerable. If
your partner works with them, and you wash her/his clothes, make

love with her/him – or even live within breathing distance of the same mill or mine – you are vulnerable too.

It's less easy to see why some people therefore put value judgements on cervical cancer as an unhygienic disease. It is no more dirty – and no less shocking – than silicosis. It certainly doesn't mean that the sufferer does not wash or care about her personal hygiene. Industrial dirt, diesel fumes and chemicals are not easily washed away; they linger on the skin and in the air. What it means is that some women's vulnerability to such things is in a special, sexual area rather than in a more easily talked about area such as the lungs.

That said, one of the factors that may lead to illness is a lack of good washing facilities. If your work place doesn't have showers, or your house doesn't have a bathroom, you are at a disadvantage. You need to make sure that you get that advantage back, and fight for a better environment.

Lack of knowledge and skill

Why include lack of knowledge and skill as factors that lead to cervical conditions? Vulnerability is not only about being undernourished or stressed. It is also about being open to attack because you have no defence.

If a woman has no knowledge of what a positive smear means or how to get one, if when she goes to get one she cannot communicate with the doctor, if she hasn't the words or the assertiveness to ask for the treatment she needs, then she is vulnerable. And this can be a factor in the development of CIN, and cancer taking a hold.

There are women without the resources to enter the health service system and fight for what they want. They range from very young women to women who are unable to speak the language of the country they are in, or are unaccustomed to medical practices and bureaucracy. Others may be too old to cope with the red tape and the waiting, or not assertive enough to ask for what they need. All of these women are vulnerable: delays can occur, treatment may be too late or inadequate. The disease develops, not because of what the woman eats, or whether she smokes, but because she cannot get the best from the system.

The problem is not confined to cervical cancer, of course. Women with other medical problems may find themselves in the same situation. Perhaps, though, we need to remember that cervical conditions in particular can make some women embarrassed, and therefore less able to cope.

Lack of medical resources

Doctors themselves can add to a woman's vulnerability by being ignorant or simply not having the time or energy to spare. Some of the women I talked to told me of doctors brushing off their inquiries about smears or follow-up treatment as 'trivial'. It can seem, when your last patient was dying, that the woman who comes with CIN 1 is wasting your time.

All too often, however, doctors are very willing to help, and it is the money and resources that are lacking. Because of lack of government funding, some women may experience difficulty in having smears more than once every few years. Once a smear is taken, the waiting time for diagnosis, and then treatment, can be alarmingly long. The condition can worsen in the interval.

Of course, this situation varies depending on the area in which you live. Well-to-do areas often have better screening programmes, bigger hospitals and better facilities, while poorer areas have long waiting lists and fewer laser machines. As always, women who are in lower-paid jobs, unemployed, or at home have less opportunity to change area, or pay for private health care services. This is responsible for yet another vulnerability.

Tobacco

Most people nowadays know that smoking makes you more vulnerable to lung cancer. Cigarette adverts tell you this clearly, in large letters. What they often don't say is that smoking also greatly increases your risk of getting cervical cancer and CIN. Smoking twenty cigarettes a day can make you seven times more vulnerable; forty cigarettes a day makes you fourteen times more vulnerable.

Smoking is harmful in a number of ways. First, it lowers your resistance to any disease or infection. In a general sense it weakens your heart and lungs, making you more likely to get ill. Also, the nicotine in cigarettes finds its way into the mucus which covers your cervix. The nicotine actually seeps through into the mucus and affects the cervical cells. Those cells, as we saw in the chapter on Facts, are constantly changing. The presence of nicotine in them destroys the immune system which keeps them healthy. So they are then more likely to change abnormally.

Very few of the women I spoke to smoked. Some of them had, but had stopped after their positive smear. Most of them agreed that smoking made them more vulnerable, although few of them saw a direct link. A few had tried to give up, and couldn't. As Lily said: 'I shouldn't be smoking I know, but at the moment (she was waiting for a further operation) I just can't stop.'

The Pill

When the contraceptive pill first came on the market, it seemed the answer to all our problems. With the arrival of the Pill came the chance for women to choose to have children, responsibly and with awareness. Now it seems that the Pill has a number of side effects. We have all heard horror stories of the Pill, and many of us have suffered our own minor horror stories of weight gain and depression. Although it is still the most reliable form of contraception, it may not, as far as women are concerned, be the 'safest', especially in relation to cervical cancer and CIN.

In the first place, the Pill can reduce our body's natural immunity to infection, making us more likely to fall ill. It can also reduce the body's ability to take in and use folic acid – and recent American work suggests that women with positive smears often have a folic acid deficiency. Next, using the Pill on its own leaves you open to catching a sexually transmitted virus or infection. As later sections of this chapter show, some doctors believe that these viruses are a factor in the development of cervical cancer and CIN. If a woman is not on the Pill, this theory goes, she or her partner usually uses a barrier form of contraception, which protects her. If she is on the Pill, usually they don't, which leaves her more vulnerable.

But does the Pill itself directly create cervical conditions which

enable cancer to develop? There is considerable evidence to suggest
that women on the Pill develop cervical problems more often than
other women.[5] On the other hand, many doctors say that the Pill is
not a factor in cervical cancer. They also point out that the risks to
women by not taking the Pill – through abortion and birth
complications – can be greater than the risks from taking the Pill.
We are faced with unclear evidence, and this means that it is easy
for people to interpret it in whichever way they want.

It is possible that doctors are influenced by the thought of what
might happen if all women turned against the Pill. Many women
would not want to stop making love spontaneously. And some
doctors imagine that, without the Pill, there would be far more
unwanted pregnancies. As Sue said: 'They don't want to mention
the Pill because it's such a nice, convenient thing.'

This seems to me to be a patronizing attitude to take towards
women. Most of us *are* able to think and choose for ourselves, and
can take responsibility for not 'getting ourselves pregnant'. (The
unwritten message in that phrase of course is that women are solely
responsible for pregnancy; but it takes two to tango.) In short, if we
believe that the Pill makes us vulnerable, we can choose not to take
it, and also choose not to get pregnant.

Sexual behaviour

There is much evidence to suggest that women's vulnerability to
cervical cancer and CIN is directly linked to heterosexual love-
making. The research started in 1842 when an Italian physician
carried out a study in which he concluded that nuns did not get
cervical cancer. Further research showed that there was a high
frequency of cervical conditions among prostitutes.

In much of the literature, therefore, one finds comments like:
'Nuns don't get it . . .', and its concomitant: 'Prostitutes do . . .'
This can build up a picture in our minds of cervical cancer as a
disease of indiscriminate sexual activity. In fact, one study in the
1950s[6] showed that some nuns do get cervical cancer, and it is now
increasingly accepted that many women attending colposcopy
clinics for treatment have had only one or two partners, often in
long-term relationships.

However, there does still seem to be a link between sexual history and a woman's vulnerability to cervical cancer. Research has shown that a high number of women with positive smears also have certain patterns of sexual behaviour.[7] The main links seem to be these:

> *The earlier a woman first has intercourse, the more vulnerable she is.*

During our teenage years, the soft cells of the vagina and cervix (columnar cells) are replaced by harder (squamous) cells more able to cope with the pressure of penetration. If penetration happens early in our lives, then these cells might not have fully formed. The softer cells can be damaged and made more vulnerable. In addition, intercourse without barrier contraception may make it more likely for a woman to catch a vulnerability-inducing virus or infection.

> *The earlier a woman has her first child the more vulnerable she is.*

This theory is based on the same idea – that early use of the cervix, before the cells are fully formed, may damage it. Also, cervical erosions occur often in women who have had children, and can make women more vulnerable. This idea is mentioned in only some of the literature available, and is not as widely accepted as other theories. However it is also not such good headline material as the next theory:

> *The more partners a woman has had, the more vulnerable she is. And the more partners her partners have had, the more vulnerable she is.*

Here again, opinions vary. Studies suggest that women with CIN and cancer often have more than one partner. Also, these women often have partners who have slept with more than one person. This would suggest that there is some sort of 'cancer trigger' that is being spread to women through men and back again. Some studies suggest that the possibility of cancer is lower when we or our partners use a barrier form of contraception like the cap or condom, and that using these methods can actually help clear up the condition.

There is a problem with such theorizing. It so easily leads to people suggesting that all women with cervical conditions have had a multitude of male partners – and value judgements being made. We can forget that it takes just one partner to create vulnerability. It can lead to our forgetting that for every woman who has 'caught' the cancer trigger, there is a man who has passed it on to her. We very quickly enter blame territory and this is very disturbing to the many, many people whose sex lives have hitherto been happy and untroubled, and who are now suddenly faced with the thought of a link between it and cervical disease.

Furthermore, the evidence is not clear-cut. Many women who have had several sexual partners never have a positive smear. Many monogamous women do, and it seems that there are many women developing CIN who have only ever had one or two male partners even if now they do not make love with men at all. Interestingly, there seems to be no correlation between frequency of love-making and vulnerability, nor with the number of children you have.

Adding fuel to the fire, there is still argument about the reasons why the number of sexual partners matters. We still don't know for certain exactly what is the possible 'cancer trigger' that is sexually transmitted. Below are listed some of the theories for what that trigger is. In every case, the research is still ongoing. Also in every case, many women who don't seem to have that particular trigger develop CIN and cancer; and many of us who do carry particular triggers remain healthy and cancer-free.

Possible sexual triggers

Sperm . One theory is that a protein substance in some sperm causes changes in the cells of the cervix. The sperm, thought to be present in certain 'high-risk' men, may be especially dangerous when it touches an unformed, maturing cervix. This fits in with the theory which states that women who make love early are more vulnerable. It also fits with the theory that the more partners a woman takes, the more at risk she is.

Cancer partners. Partners of men who develop cancer of the genitals often seem to later develop CIN and cervical cancer. It follows therefore, that the more partners you have, the higher the probability that you will have one partner who later develops cancer and, according to this theory, the greater the risk to yourself. The evidence for this theory is, however, contradictory.

Infections. It has been suggested that sexually transmitted infections can decrease your natural immune system, making you more likely to catch any disease. In particular, they can also increase your vulnerability to cancer. Women with positive smears have been found to have a high incidence of thrush, gardnerella and trichomoniasis.

Infections that cause a discharge may also make it easier for the wart virus to develop in the vagina. The wart virus grows more easily when discharge is present – and as we shall see later, is seen by some to be connected with cancer and CIN.

The herpes virus. The herpes virus is currently being investigated, because many women with positive smears have this virus. In particular, a current theory suggests that the herpes virus and the wart virus together can create vulnerable conditions on the cervix. However not all medical professionals agree on this yet.

The wart virus. In the past few years, there has been much publicity of the wart virus. 'HPV-16 almost certainly causes cervical cancer', shrieked one headline.

As mentioned in Chapter 8, there are a group of viruses which cause warts in various parts of the body, including the sexual parts. But even when there are no warts to be seen, the wart virus may be present on the genitals. It will be passed on from partner to partner, and of course the higher the number of partners, the greater the chance of catching the wart virus.

But does wart virus make cancer more likely? Some research has suggested that certain varieties of the wart virus cause changes in the cells on the cervix, making them grow uncontrollably.[8] Some wart viruses seem to be responsible for a new, fast developing form of cancer. Other theories suggest that the wart virus can only create cancer cells when other factors, such as the herpes virus, are present.

However, not all experts agree with the research – and even more of them disagree with the interpretation.[9] (The only long-term studies of the effect of the relevant wart viruses on cervical conditions are not due to end until 1998.) Firstly, not all women who have CIN or cervical cancer have these wart viruses. So there must be other factors involved. Also, many women who have the wart virus don't develop either warts or CIN. Some estimates say that 70 per cent of the population have the wart virus anyway, so it would not be surprising that many of the CIN women tested seemed to have the virus.[10]

There have also been studies which show that, in cases where both the wart virus and CIN are present, even when the wart virus is not cured, most women treated for CIN do not get CIN again. If a relation had existed between the two, it could reasonably be supposed that the CIN would have re-occurred.[11]

A final theory is just now coming to light. The wart virus may create conditions on the cervix which on a smear test read as advanced CIN 3. But these conditions are reversible, and not at all the same as true CIN changes. We simply don't have enough information to say whether this theory is true.

So in the end, the situation is unclear. At the time of going to press it seems likely that using barrier contraception reduces your vulnerability to CIN and cancer, but why and exactly how is not evident.

What is probably clear to you at this stage is this: if there is a link between sexual behaviour and your positive smear, you may need to stop and think. Other chapters of this book look at the very real concerns these issues raise for us as women, our relationships with our partners and with society. For in this area, cervical cancer does not just affect our health – it touches our partnerships, our morality and our self-esteem. In particular, the leap from the statement 'sexual behaviour may be linked with cervical cancer' to 'promiscuity causes cervical cancer' is one which we should all be wary of. For the first statement may be a fact; the second statement can never be anything but a biased value judgement.

Stress

Stress has always been identified as one of the things that stops us being healthy. We get ill more easily, we throw off disease more slowly. Many of the women I spoke to mentioned stress as a factor. They talked of being overworked or worried. And they told me how one of the first things they did after hearing that they had a positive smear was to try to cut down their work load and worry less. 'I've always been a worrier,' said one woman. 'Now I know I must take things easy – I have no choice.'

Past experiences

As I interviewed the women who had contacted me, I noticed a strange pattern emerging. It was not one that has ever been mentioned in relation to positive smears, however it was clearly present. The pattern was this: many of the women I spoke to who had had positive smears had also had in their lives some trauma attached to sexuality or fertility.

Two of the women I spoke to had been raped. Several had had abortions. Many spoke of traumatic relationships: 'It was as if I was being punished for having an abortion'; 'My punishment . . . for the abortion and for people I'd slept with in the past'; 'I always linked my CIN with sleeping with someone when I knew I didn't want to . . .'

I wonder at this. I would not want to suggest that a traumatic incident in early life triggered CIN or cancer or that the stress of early trauma created a vulnerability in which cancer or CIN could develop. And yet the women I spoke to saw a link, even if only in their minds, which caused them pain and guilt. So although doctors and researchers are concentrating on what they think causes cervical disease, I would like to point out that many women make entirely different mental links, which affect the way they think and feel. It would be helpful if doctors were aware of this.

Miscellaneous

Some women I talked to rejected all the theories. Some considered they were just unlucky. Some thought it was just 'one of those things': 'I weighed up all these causes and thought it might not be any of those. So I didn't worry about it too much.' (Rachel).

Others came up with their own, special theories: 'I have a skin condition (psoriasis) in which cells multiply. It seemed as if CIN was the same thing,' said Jane G. 'I'd recently been suppressing a lot of emotion – it was a way of getting rid of all the tension I had down there,' thought Hilda.

None of these things are seriously mentioned in the leaflets or the articles by professionals. Yet they may ring true for you and if they do, perhaps they are more relevant to you than all the research on smoking, and diet and viruses.

Knowing your vulnerabilities

In the end, whatever it is that creates your particular vulnerability is specifically yours. Jane G. said: 'My illness was my illness and to do with me,' and that seems to sum it up. Certainly there is a great deal of evidence which points to links between certain factors and the positive smear. Smoking, the Pill, sexual behaviour all seem to be things to consider carefully.

Considering these factors, you might, perhaps for the first time in your life, have looked at what makes you vulnerable – not only to cervical cancer, but also to a host of other illnesses and diseases. You may now have to rethink your attitude to many things in your life – to partners, to contraception, to yourself.

You may, on consideration, decide to change nothing. But now at least you have some idea of the odds.

10

FEELING GOOD ABOUT YOURSELF

'I was dealing with it very well . . . it was me, and I was dealing with it . . .' (Julie)

Some illnesses come and go and leave you as you were before. You still have no less, or no more liking for yourself than you ever had. You don't (usually) break your arm and spend time feeling guilty that you were clumsy enough to fall over.

Having a positive smear can be very different. I did speak to women who saw it as just another illness. But for surprisingly many, it was 'not the same as a cut on your arm'. There are hidden and not-so-hidden messages surrounding the condition, hinting that maybe this time it is your fault, or causing you to think that you shouldn't feel quite so good about yourself as you did before, or that women in general are to blame.

If we are to recover fully from a cervical condition, and if we are, socially, to avoid victim-blame, then we need to look at these messages carefully and work out ways to deal with them.

Messages from the past

Where do we get the messages about our own worth? The foundations are laid early on in life: some of these messages may lie dormant for years, then suddenly reappear, precipitated by an event in your life. So if at some time in the past, you got the message that making love was wrong, if when you were small you were told that a doctor was a god-like creature – then these messages may still be with you. They are probably all the stronger because they've been with you for longer. You may believe them without question.

Then they are reactivated by cues from your present situation. If, like Emma, you get a doctor who 'made me feel in the way', then the chances are that this will increase any emotional vulnerability you already have, making you feel even more vulnerable.

Many of the women I spoke to admitted that before the smear, they had had negative feelings about themselves – their health, their sexuality, their emotions. The experience of the positive smear set everything off again. As Judith said: 'I was raped when I was sixteen and the positive smear brought it all back; I had to go through it all again.' This is a very dramatic example. But even a slight lack of self-esteem, common to most women in our society, can be intensified by the news of a positive smear.

The cues

What are the cues that trigger negative feelings? They can be very personal ones; your partner's reaction, for example: 'There's nothing the matter with you – what are you going on about . . .' Many women found that if people who were close thought worse of them for having a positive smear, they began to think worse of themselves.

But the cues can come from much less intimate sources. If a doctor speaks to you in a patronizing manner; if a consultant says that the fact that you sleep with your boyfriend could have created your problem, it can be enough to set you off on a spiral of self-blame. It's important to realize that often, when women are dealing with medical professionals, they start by believing that 'the doctor is always right'. And if s/he is right about the disease and the treatment, then s/he must be right in his/her judgement of you.

Finally, you can be affected by 'what the papers say'. The press, television and radio are often very supportive of the cancer cause. However, they are also tempted by a good headline to create stories that blame. They seize on the theory that women who have more than one partner seem more likely to develop cancer and CIN – and they add on words like 'promiscuous'. Is it any wonder that we feel guilty when faced with publicity like this?

Many of the women I spoke to admitted feeling bad about themselves at some time after hearing the positive smear news.

Sometimes this self-doubt lasted minutes, in some cases months. Frances said that she still, a year later, didn't feel as confident as she used to before it happened.

Self-blame

And what are the things that we worry about – what particular issues carry all these feelings of self-blame? There seemed to be a number of them; here is how women expressed them:

'I'm not healthy'

Some women felt bad about getting ill in the first place. Particularly if they'd been very healthy before, they thought that somehow their bodies had let them down. Rachel's very perceptive consultant commented that: 'many women who thought they were healthy get their self-esteem knocked when it happens.'

Once 'it' has happened, if you don't get better on your own, you can feel even worse. Several of my interviewees, particularly those who believed in the power of the mind over the body, were concerned if their efforts at self-cure failed. Julia was 'a bit disappointed as I'd hoped I could make it go away.'

It is certainly true that having a positive smear reminds many of us of our mortality. It is even more striking because in most cases there are no symptoms, no visible signs, to tell us that something is wrong. And as one woman put it: 'I realize that I can never be totally certain of my health again.'

It may also mean that we simply adapt to this new awareness of our vulnerability. Now that we are aware of it, and can take steps, the vulnerability itself can actually be neutralized. Before, when we were unaware, we were doing nothing about it. Now at least we can take action.

'I'm dirty'

As we explained in the chapter on Causes, poor living and working conditions can make you more vulnerable to cervical disease. Industrial dirt, diesel fumes and lack of washing facilities can create just the right conditions for its development.

For some reason, this fact often gets interpreted as meaning that cervical cancer is a disease of women who are 'dirty'. And lots of women take this message on board. Julie 'imagined this tacky, dirty, ugly, black-looking cervix . . .' and not surprisingly felt bad about it.

This is one myth we can dispel at once. Cervical cancer is not a disease of unhygienic women; it is a disease of an unhygienic environment.

'It's my fault'

This was a common reaction. Women convinced themselves that there must be a chain of cause and effect and they were therefore the cause. Surely, this thinking went, if we have this condition, it must be due to something that we have done.

Two women spoke about their abortions, and made an emotional link between the self-blame they were feeling now and the guilt they felt when they had had the abortion: 'I've really regretted that, and the threat of a cone biopsy, which at the time I thought might affect my ability to have children, seemed the worst thing that could happen to me,' said one.

Many women mentioned feeling uneasy about sex. There is a creeping fear that if you hadn't slept with him, then you might never have got . . . that infection, that virus, that CIN, that cancer. So of course it is *your* fault.

In practical terms, remember that talking about fault is inaccurate. The fact that you have a cervical condition is not anyone's fault. Even if there is a connection between sex and cervical cancer, you did not create it. You merely caught it from someone else, who caught it from someone else. You are a victim, not someone to be blamed. Remember too that your cervical condition may well have been caused by one of the many other contributing factors. No one can ever tell you that it is your sex life that is to blame – or that it is your fault.

Often though, the guilty emotion isn't even based on the knowledge that there may be a direct link between sex and cervical cancer. For there is still a feeling abroad that it is bad to make love, that in some way, if anything bad happens that has a sexual link, then we are getting our just deserts.

You may or may not regret having slept with your partners. If you do regret any of your partnerships, then that is most likely due to the relationship you had with that person. For a doctor, or anyone else, to ask you to start regretting a relationship because now, months or years later, you have an illness of a sexual part of your body, is unacceptable. Don't give in to it.

'People will think I'm promiscuous'

This self-doubt is not an idle fear. Women like Linda worried that 'people will point a finger at me . . .' because they'd heard other people say that cervical cancer means you sleep around. Some women were actually confronted by friends and relatives: 'My husband's mother rang me one evening to say that she'd heard you only get it if you're promiscuous. I said to her – I've only slept with one man and that's your son,' reported one woman.

You may have had one sexual partner, or several sexual partners. That is a fact and is indisputable. But to comment negatively on this fact is a value judgement. It is someone else's view, and it does not have to be yours. Sleeping with X number of partners is a fact. To define this as 'promiscuous' is a value judgement, and demeaning to you and your relationships. If you are happy with the number of people you have slept with, then no one else has the right to comment, let alone criticize.

So don't fall for it when you read the newspapers, or switch on the television. Don't fall for it when colleagues joke, or friends insinuate. Above all, don't fall for it if partners blame. If you don't fall for it, agree with it, or collude with it, then gradually people will learn that it is not to be done. Facts are one thing, value judgements are another.

'I might not be able to have children'

Some women I spoke to, particularly if they were young and had not yet started a family, felt bad because they were afraid their ability to have children had been affected. You can feel very down if that aspect of your womanhood is important to you and is under threat – and your negative feelings could well rebound on yourself.

If you have had a hysterectomy, then obviously childbearing is impossible. And if this is so, you may feel understandably depressed. Hysterectomy support groups could help you recover your self-esteem and work through your sense of loss.

If you have not had a hysterectomy, it is unlikely that your child-bearing ability will be affected. Occasionally a cone biopsy may make having children more tricky, which is why it is more often used for older women who have completed their families. If you are worried about this and have been advised to have a cone biopsy, then check with your doctor whether you really do need one.

Treatments such as laser or diathermy will almost certainly have no adverse effect on your ability to bear children. On the contrary, the removal of abnormal cells and the consequent improvement of your general health, will probably have also improved your chances of having a healthy family.

'I might die'

As mentioned before, death from cervical conditions is extremely rare. But this doesn't mean to say that no woman is ever afraid. If you do feel frightened, then you are not alone; a large proportion of women, even with CIN conditions, were afraid at some point during the process.

The thing to do is to accept that you have a right to be frightened and that being so doesn't mean you are weak. Then remember that there is in all probability no reason for you to be so; the overwhelming majority of women with a positive smear do not have cancer, and the overwhelming majority of those with cancer survive to a ripe old age. If you are worried, check with your doctor about the seriousness of your condition; tell him you would prefer to know the truth and cope with it than be denied the possibility of coping by not knowing.

'I feel dependent on the doctors'

A lot of women's lack of confidence sprang from their relationship with the doctors dealing with their case. We'll be looking more closely at the relationship between patients and doctors in Chapter 13. For now, let's look briefly at what can happen with medical professionals that reduces a woman's self esteem.

A woman can feel dependent on the professionals, doctors and nurses, and often the way procedures are set up encourages this feeling. Having to undress and then lie in a vulnerable position to be examined also make us feel powerless.

The attitude of doctors can make things worse. I know that many doctors are caring human beings who respect and admire the women they treat. But far too many of my interviewees had come into contact with doctors who were not like this. There were many reports of questions going unanswered, and there were also many complaints about doctors being patronizing or 'talking down' to their patients. When women tried to discuss treatment, they were often met with an unwillingness to accept the possibility that they have any say in the matter.

Happily, many of my interviewees came to their own decisions and voted with their feet. Some changed doctors, others fought for, and got, the treatment they wanted. So they were able to overcome their feelings of dependence and powerlessness. They replaced them, not with feelings of power over the doctors, but with a feeling of being respected and involved in the process of their own health.

'Maybe I shouldn't be making all this fuss'

Many women cope beautifully with having a positive smear, whether that means cancer or CIN. But we don't all respond like this. Many of us panic even before we know we have a serious illness, and get very emotional if we find out we have. In particular, I found many women with CIN who had been frightened, angry, guilty and sad while at the same time knowing that their condition was not serious and that they would soon be well.

Sometimes feeling all these emotions can seem self-indulgent: 'You feel wicked, going on about it for so long . . .' said Anna, who had a CIN condition. Three months after her operation, she burst into tears when her GP asked her how she was. The doctor, understanding what was happening to her, listened for a while and then put her in touch with a counselling service.

Sometimes the response is not quite so positive. Linda's husband commented: 'What's all the fuss about – you haven't got cancer,' and this can be the attitude of many partners, friends and doctors. There is a mixed message here: while on the one hand you need to take the condition seriously, have regular smears, and take precautions against it deteriorating, on the other you have to bear in mind that your condition is nevertheless minor. Though it might not seem minor to you.

If you have to have more aggressive treatment, you can still feel just as confused – and could get the same response from people who are trying to help. 'They kept saying "It's nothing" but it wasn't nothing to me,' said Diana about her hysterectomy. If you know that you have a serious disease, you need two things: firstly some hope that it is going to be all right, and secondly the opportunity to cry and scream and shout if you feel like it, because all this is happening to you.

Guilt about these feelings can be eased. You can ask people not to tell you 'it's nothing', and ask them to support you while you accept that what is happening does affect you. You can also remember that one of the reasons they want to reassure you is that your fears and your anger make them feel bad; they are simply protecting themselves against their own emotions by asking you to dampen down yours.

Feeling good about yourself

Lots of women coped with their positive smear experience and gained extra strength from it. They were able to look back afterwards and feel good about what they had done.

Sue said that after her hysterectomy, she often reminded herself what she had to be glad of in her life: 'With a little formula . . . I'm still alive, I don't have periods anymore . . .' She, and many of the other women, talked about 'coming through it all', and how they felt that it was something to be proud of.

Perhaps you think that being asked to find positive things in an illness is rather too much of a challenge for many women. If so, all I can say is that in that case many of us have a remarkable capacity for rising to the challenge.

Many women used the experience to get more in touch with what they needed. Being ill and feeling vulnerable seemed to help them to realize that they had to take better care of themselves. Many improved their diet, or their exercise habits. Many gave up smoking. One woman began taking holidays for the first time, and almost all said that they had recognized a need to relax and lead a less stressful life. Some reported changing to forms of contraception they felt were more healthy.

In the same way, having a positive smear helped women to get in touch with what they wanted. Many women had to do this in order to survive. They fought hard to get the doctors they wanted or the treatment they wanted. One woman refused to agree to a hysterectomy until after an exploratory operation. Another went on an assertiveness course to help her cope. Many of the women who went through the positive smear experience learned, as Jane G. did, that: 'We can find out what it is we need, and we can make a choice and get it.'

Many women came through the experience not only with more strength for themselves, but also with more strength for others. When it is all over, and you begin to have time for other people again, then the very fact that you have been through it could mean that you want to help other women. This is a way of feeling good about yourself, too.

'I can help other people because I was helped. I feel good about that,' says Diana, who now writes positive smear advice leaflets for her local gynaecological clinic. Lily Hopkins went on television to plead the cause of women in her area whose smear results had been wrongly diagnosed. Jane B. has set up a telephone network in her area for women with cervical cancer. There are ways to feel good – and to feel good about yourself – even on the worst days.

11

BUILDING YOUR OWN SUPPORT SYSTEM

My sister was invaluable . . . she just wouldn't let me give
up. (Heather)

You may think of yourself as already being part of a wide social
network. You may be a loner, and getting support is not something
you find easy. But you will handle the positive smear experience
better if you find out just what sort of support system you need, and
then get it for yourself.

What sort of support system do you need?

A support system can be many things. Some women mentioned
wanting sources of information, to help them in their discussions
with doctors. And if this is true for you, then good links with local
libraries, or the district women's centre or health centre will be all
you need. You might need the support of another person here too:
Heather's sister 'marched me round to all the libraries to follow up
references.'

You may need very practical help, such as child care while you
attend appointments or someone to buy your food while you are
convalescing after a cone biopsy. It is a good idea to sit down at each
stage in the experience, and work out exactly what you need and
how. One woman arranged a rota of friends to take her for
radiotherapy; they took turns to collect her and bring her back, and
then settled her in bed for a rest and a hot drink.

For most of us, support also means being able to talk about what
is happening. You might need an occasional chat, in order just to
begin to assimilate the experience. You might on occasions need

someone with you for a longer period of time, to allow you to feel safe and cared for. On my return from my operation, a friend stayed with me overnight – not so much because of my physical condition, but because I just felt weepy.

It is worth asking yourself what you particularly need from people in the way of emotional support, for we are all different. Julie 'needed to feel I was coping on my own'. Judith 'told everyone'. Some women like to feel that they are coping by forgetting that it is happening and doing things that take their mind off the problem – others feel the need to be allowed to cry and get angry when they want to. So stop and think just what your needs are, at various times, and with various people: to be held, talked to, allowed to talk, supported in feeling your emotions, distracted from the problems, told 'it's OK', told 'it's OK to be frightened.'

Who can support you?

The support system that you want might not be full of people. You might prefer to cope on your own. But if you do need people support, whom do you need? You may get help from parents, from children, from family, from friends, from colleagues – and from professional helpers of all kinds. I have not included here the particular support you can get from your intimate partner, because getting support from a partner can often raise problems – and opportunities – that just don't occur in other situations. Chapter 12 covers this in more detail.

Family support can often be the strongest and most binding kind. When you have known someone from birth, you are likely to want to fight to keep them healthy and happy. Viki and Anna, mother and daughter, both had CIN conditions within a very short time of each other: 'Anna was with me through the whole thing and she was very helpful,' said Viki. Heather's sister commented: 'I was determined to support her well.'

Friends, on the other hand, can give much more objective support. They can tell you, where perhaps your mother wouldn't, when you are panicking too much and when you are not standing up for yourself. One friend I had came round when I heard the news, armed with a bottle of wine and a calm: 'Now, I've just seen a television programme, and it said that what you've got is totally curable. So stop whingeing.'

Colleagues are perhaps the least concerned; they may not know you well, or be able to appreciate your emotions. Also, mixing emotions or illnesses with the work situation may be frowned upon. Few of the women I talked to felt able to confide in colleagues or use them as part of an ongoing support system, although one woman told a story of a delightful female boss who allowed her limitless time off for hospital appointments.

It is possibly most difficult to know how to relate to children. They do give support, by being there and by giving affection. But it's difficult to tell them what is going on – and they could be upset that Mummy seems absent-minded all of a sudden, or keeps having to go off and leave them with friends. Few of the women I talked to had told their children what was happening because their families were too young. Only Jane B. had told her teenage daughter that she was starting a cancer support group, and received the ultimate accolade: 'I think you could do it, Mum!'

The above are all people you will have known before the positive smear. However you can also choose to get some of your support from people who are strangers to you – professional support people such as counsellors who are trained and experienced in talking to people with just your sort of worries. You don't need to have a serious illness to seek professional support. Many women I spoke to with CIN 1 had rung up a health or cancer support agency and had been given information and attention from the helpers there.

Remember too that if you do seek professional aid, you aren't in any way rejecting the care your family and friends offer you. You may in fact be helping them to cope – and also giving yourself more of the type of support you need – because perhaps the people who are closest to you are the very ones who can't support you. If you are seriously ill, they may be too upset themselves to give you the help you need. If you have a minor condition, they may shrug it off, thinking that you are simply making a fuss. For remember that some people are uneasy with illness, emotion and sexuality. Also, your distress might trigger their distress and make them too upset to be useful. Counsellors, outside your situation, are not subject to these temptations.

Let's look then at some of the things that might stop the people around you from giving you really good support.

Blocks to support

Embarrassment

Firstly, you may find it quite difficult to confide, particularly in older members of your family, about what is happening to you. Your mother, father and older relatives may be so different from you in their attitudes, beliefs and ways of helping that you'd really rather not say anything to them. 'I couldn't tell my parents,' said more than one woman.

Why can't you confide in other people? Very often it is because of the stigma attached to a sexually-linked disease. More than one woman had heard her parents repeat stories about 'promiscuity and the smear test'. Anna recounts: 'I didn't tell my colleagues because I'd heard various derogatory comments about women with positive smears.' Knowing that it might not be easy to explain all the mixed messages that exist around the issue, you may choose not to tell anyone, particularly if your condition is not serious.

If you do tell people, then be prepared for a variety of responses. You may have to face talk about promiscuity or challenges to your sexual life. If you can, explain to people who give you this sort of reaction that the hype about multiple sexual partners just isn't true. Even sleeping with one man – which is something every Mum has done – will put you at risk. Janet reported that her mother, who was very supportive in many ways, commented: ' "I've never had it. Why have you got it?" I thought – it's because you're lucky, Mum.'

Fear

Equally, both relatives and friends will often find it difficult to cope with the possibility of your being seriously ill; they may panic unnecessarily. If it is clear that you have cancer, they might be so distressed at the thought of losing you that they prefer not to talk about it: 'I couldn't talk to my family because they didn't want to be reminded of it,' says Sue.

Even if it isn't clear, they may be so paralysed by the thought that they find it hard to handle: 'I knew your parents had both died of cancer recently,' said one of my close friends, 'so when you had a positive smear, I just thought: "Oh, God, it's happened again", and the thought was very hard to handle.'

Lack of understanding

A final block to really getting the support you want may be that you feel unable to talk to someone who hasn't already had the condition. You imagine that they can't begin to understand what it is like. In some cases your imagination is correct – people who haven't been through it might not be able to realize what you are feeling: 'I don't know anyone in my circle of friends who has it . . . I haven't told them,' said Frances.

On the other hand, many other people have been ill, have felt frightened, have suffered in similar ways to you – even if they haven't had a cervical condition. So don't draw back from asking simply because you are, as one woman put it, 'afraid their guts may turn'.

Helping and being helped

In fact, for many women support meant talking to others in the same situation. And this is a very real option in building your support system. Contacting other women who have had positive smears has two advantages. It means that you are always talking to someone who understands, and it means you are helping while at the same time being helped.

It also means that women are helping themselves and each other; this process can have amazing results. Lily's support group, set up after a misdiagnosis of smear tests in Liverpool, went on to gain national TV coverage and compensatory legal action. So it seems relevant to deal at length in this chapter with how to set up women's networks which can support us in a very special way.

Networking

Many of the women I spoke to had used their experience to communicate and exchange ideas with others. Some of them had used support groups mentioned in the Resource section – The Hysterectomy Support Group and various cancer support groups seemed particularly helpful. It seems, though, that there are very few groups specifically for women who have just had a positive smear. In response to this, four of the women I interviewed had set up support groups and telephone networks to provide on the spot help and support when it is most needed. Their groups met regularly; their telephone network operated when and where it was needed.

It should be remembered, however, that different women have different needs from such a network, in that their illnesses differ. One woman may need counselling after she has heard she has cancer; another may be deeply distressed at having CIN 1. The problems of someone struggling to accept that she has the wart virus and a CIN condition may be very different from those of a woman who has just completed radiotherapy.

So in some ways, the more you can specify who your group is for, the better it will work. A network for women with cervical cancer, a network for women after hysterectomies, a network for women with CIN – all of these will bring together women with the same sorts of problem and in need of the same sorts of help. You may find, of course, that the number of women who respond in your area is so small that you need to widen your scope to include all types of cervical problem.

A second thing to remember is that most positive smear women will have their condition for no more than a year, and probably a lot less. Their need is for help and support from the time they know they have a positive smear up to the time just after their treatment. This has particular repercussions for support groups. If a group meets once a month, then allowing for holidays and absences, each woman will attend on average a maximum of seven times. So it isn't surprising that many support groups come to an end because women stop coming, or because there is such a fast turnover that everyone feels uncomfortable.

Running a telephone network

In order to set up a telephone network, you will probably need a central organizer who will take the names and numbers of women who are interested in talking to other women. The most active organizational system I found was that based at the Women's Health and Reproductive Rights Information Centre. When women ring with cervical problems, they are asked if they would be willing to talk to others in the same position. If so, their names, addresses, telephone numbers and a short description of their condition is noted down. If necessary, and if the woman prefers, just a first name and phone number can be taken. They are then asked if they would like to talk to someone, and if so, their situation is matched with that of another woman on the network, and the two are put in touch with each other. Being on the network doesn't mean that you spend half your time helping others – in the seven months I've been involved, I've only been rung once. But it does mean that a woman who needs to talk has immediate access to someone who can give them a little support, confidentially and often even anonymously.

Running a support group

A support group needs a lot more resources to set up. You need a meeting place and a date that is regular enough for women to know when to turn up. You usually need someone to facilitate the discussion each time, otherwise participants can feel that their needs are not being met. Many groups arrange for a different woman to take on this role each time, and invite guest speakers such as doctors or pathologists to give their viewpoint. Be careful, though, of falling into the trap of 'bowing to the experts'.

Remember that support groups are a real chance for women to start believing that their experiences are important. It is crucial to allocate a considerable part of each meeting to 'going round the circle', letting each woman give an account of where she is in the process, what has been happening to her since the last meeting, and what her needs are at present. You will find that you don't need to 'set a topic' – the women themselves will talk about what they need to talk about. All the group needs to do is to make sure no one hogs the limelight, and that no one criticizes anyone else for what they say. Ideally, this should be a time for being able to talk freely and openly without fear of rejection.

There is a fear, both for women in support groups and those who think of telephone counselling, that somebody you are with will break down completely and you won't be able to handle it. This can happen, but it rarely does. Because human beings are good at self-preservation, and if you feel uneasy – or your support group doesn't feel safe – then women won't let go of their emotions completely. They just won't want to do it. My own experience is that if a woman does feel safe enough to cry, or to talk about her experiences in a very deep way, then the whole group feels better. Each woman can learn something from that.

The book *In Our Own Hands*, by Sheila Ernst and Lucy Goodison (The Women's Press, 1982), has some excellent information about setting up groups of all kinds. Some of the suggestions for games or 'ice-breakers' can be very valuable, particularly if a group knows each other well.

Remember that support groups can suffer from a rapidly changing clientele, so it is a good idea to have an anchor person, who opens her house once a month and is always there to start things off.

Publicizing networks

No telephone or group network will get off the ground unless people know about it. If you do decide to start one, then here are some helpful hints.

Contact your Community Health Council for the names of women's groups and health centres. Try also to find out the names of GPs in your area. Then prepare a simple poster giving the name of the network, a few words about what it does, a contact name and number. If you can, get copies put up in doctors' surgeries, health centres, and anywhere where women with positive smears may go, and you will find the word spreading. Add to this publicity by placing free ads in local news-sheets, district magazines, women's centre papers.

If you want to go more public, then contact your local newspaper and radio station. They are often glad to include a mention of your project on an afternoon programme aimed at women. Suggest to them that they interview someone (perhaps you) involved in the network who can give an idea of what it does and who it is aimed at.

Tell an anecdote or two to convince women that they are not alone in how they feel. And make sure you include your telephone number. If the interview is recorded, stand by your phone afterwards. If it is live, then either get another member of the network to be by the phone – or rush home as soon as you can. 'I got twenty-five phone calls the evening after my interview,' said Lily, 'and the phone didn't stop ringing for days.'

Support systems – what next?

It would be wonderful if 'the system' were more aware of the need for support systems for positive smear women. The reasons it is not vary widely.

Some of the medical and social work professionals I talked to were all too aware of the need for support. Many had formed hysterectomy groups within their hospitals, and often gave informal and highly effective counselling to every woman undergoing treatment. Your GP, if s/he knows you, may already be giving you this sort of support.

However, some of the professionals I talked to just didn't seem to know the need existed. They either hadn't talked to women who were upset, or thought that these women were in a very small minority. Some knew of the need, but had neither the time, the energy or the funding to give priority to support above 'treatment'. I worry that perhaps they are ignoring the fact that, with the right support, treatment would be more effective or even (heretical thought) just not necessary.

Some professionals were simply not interested in such things as formal support groups. They worried that they would consist, as one doctor said, of women 'sitting round panicking each other'. I agree there is a danger of our getting swept away by each other's distress. But there is an equal danger of our sitting on the distress so long that it overwhelms us, or of accepting that only doctors can help us, and failing to realize that we as women can help ourselves in more informal ways.

On balance, I feel that any form of positive support that women can get for themselves or offer for each other will, in both the short and the long term, do nothing but good.

12

INTIMATE RELATIONSHIPS

> I'm Emma's best friend . . . if I hadn't have been, it would
> have all been so much easier. (Alain, Emma's husband)

Of all the areas of importance that women talked about to me
through many interviews, one of the key ones was that of intimate
relationships. 'When you touch your cervix, you touch your heart,'
as Jacqui said.

So this chapter looks at all aspects of the intimate relationship as
it is affected by the positive smear experience. How do we feel
about our partners after a positive smear? What do partners really
feel when we are going through our experience of the condition?
How can we work together to make the experience a positive one
for the relationship?

Setting the framework

But what is your intimate relationship? For the purposes of this
chapter, I am assuming that it involves sex. I know that many
people who regard themselves as having an intimate relationship,
many people who see themselves as partners, don't sleep together.
Where cervical conditions are concerned, however, I found that
there were particular issues, and particular challenges, to be found
within relationships that involved sex.

The main focus of these rewards and challenges is bound to be
the relationship or relationships you are in at the time you experience the positive smear process. Most of the women I talked to had
one central relationship at that time, although a few women had
more than one. And this in itself can cause problems: 'I didn't want

my husband to be there when I was treated, I wanted my lover to be there,' said Evelyn. But for the general purposes of this chapter, I shall speak as if you have one current relationship.

I shall also usually use the word 'he' to describe your partner. Women who have positive smears may have female lovers, but what I found was that whether we are lesbian or heterosexual, it is the male–female link that creates many of the negative feelings linked with cervical cancer.

The women's experience

Having a positive smear puts women in a very vulnerable position. In particular, as I have already pointed out, it makes us stop and think about sex, and so naturally about our sexual, intimate relationships. Of the women I talked to, a minority felt that their partners had no place in what was happening, and that this was their own experience, to be gone through alone. Most of them saw it as an experience that involved their partner; some saw it as an issue between their partner and themselves.

Abandonment

Very many women felt sad and angry at the way their partners reacted to their condition. The cry again and again was: 'He didn't seem to realize what I was going through.' We are talking here about the way partners behaved – and the fact that it was often not what women wanted. Here are some sample complaints: 'He was away all the time'; 'He needed me to comfort him'; 'I don't think he believed how serious it was'; 'He didn't want to know'; 'He didn't want to talk about it'; 'He built a brick wall'; 'He refused to read any of the literature'; 'He didn't come with me to the hospital – and that finished our relationship.'

It was not all negative. There were also many women who said their partners were supportive and gave them what they needed. Many of the women quoted above had stable relationships that in other ways were totally satisfactory. Some women, in fact, wanted less support, not more, as it made them feel dependent and weak to be over-protected.

However there did seem to be a pattern of men seemingly not 'understanding . . . listening . . . taking it seriously.' If you feel that this is your partner's response, you are not alone. It does not mean that your relationship is at an end – as we shall see when we look at what some men said, it doesn't even mean that your partner doesn't understand you. Nevertheless, you may start to panic, feeling that just at the time when you need him most, he's not there for you. As we shall see later, you may well be right – but not for the reasons that you suspect.

Blame

'Often, when you hear that you have a positive smear, your first thought is: Who did I get this from?' as one woman put it. At the time of going to press, the link between sexual contact and cervical cancer is not clear, nor is it proven. Equally, it may not be the particular trigger that made you vulnerable. It is newsworthy, however, and sufficiently publicized so that many women immediately jump to the conclusion that they 'caught' their cervical condition from a man.

Many women made this connection, and spoke scathingly of partners because of it. Some blamed past partners: 'We split up two and a half years ago . . . I feel this [the CIN condition] is the result of him having other relationships which I hadn't known about at the time,' said Rosemary. Some blamed present partners: 'The first thing I said when I heard was, "I'll kill him",' said one woman. Some women felt confused and uncertain: 'I don't blame him – but I want to know what caused it,' said Linda.

Many women of course, saw this as absolutely not an issue: 'We didn't enter into that,' said Julie, 'I know that isn't an issue for us . . .' They knew that there was a possibility of a kickback from previous relationships, but it wasn't relevant to their present security. In any case, as one woman said, 'I've also had relationships before ours; it might have been me rather than him.'

It is totally understandable that if your partner has passed a virus on to you, such as the wart virus, that you should be upset by this. It is not a pleasant thing to have. Mary, who did catch the wart virus from her boyfriend, was 'very angry as well as hurt.' And if your partner does have an infection or virus and is unwilling to have it treated, then you are right to be angry. It is also understandable if you are hurt by your partner's past and present sexual history. If we are not the only sexual partner in our man's life, then that may also provoke strong feeling. So if your cervical condition reminds you of the fact that your partner has slept with other women, then don't be surprised if you start to feel negative.

Remember, however, that it is never certain that your partner's past or present sexual history has any direct link with your particular current condition. Many women have relationships without developing cervical cancer; many men have relationships without their partners developing it. There are many vulnerability factors that can band together to affect you, of which sexually-caused vulnerability is only one.

Political anger

Some women who spoke to me placed the responsibility on men in a much wider sense. They felt that men in general were to blame for irresponsible sexual behaviour which might be spreading the 'cancer trigger'. They felt that in the arena of sexual politics, men were the oppressors again by inflicting yet another sexual disease on women.

Arguments for and against the 'cancer trigger' theory apart, it seems to be a big leap of judgement to say that men are therefore to blame for cervical cancer. Certainly if there is a direct link between sexual activity and cervical abnormality, the current tendency to blame women is not the answer. Yet neither, I think, is blaming men. Men should assume equal responsibility for taking pre-cautions, not only against cervical cancer but against all forms of sexually transmitted disease, as well as against pregnancy. Men, like women, should guard against these things by being responsible in safe sex, and by working to enhance and prolong good, fulfilling relationships.

However, to say, as some people do while championing women's causes, that cervical cancer is men's fault, is too easy a route. If the cancer trigger is a virus, and a man has caught it, then who has he caught it from? It is more than likely that he has caught it from another woman, who in turn has caught it from a man, who in turn . . . If the 'cancer trigger' is not a virus, but is rogue sperm, then it is neither men's fault for having rogue sperm, nor women's fault for being attracted to men.

Unless we women are to give up all forms of sex involving penile penetration, then we must take equal responsibility for wanting that particular form of love-making, and – now that we know the facts – equal responsibility for the dangers that may involve.

Guilt

If an ex-partner of yours is now going out with someone new, this can lead to further bad feelings. My ex-lover's new girlfriend developed CIN 2 and had laser treatment. I was tempted to believe that he had caught something from me and passed 'it' on to his new girlfriend – and that it was my fault.

If you are scared of this, and you have just had a positive smear result, then you may feel you ought to mention it to your ex-partner. But remember that it is up to him and his new partner to make their own decisions about what they do; whether they use barrier contraception, whether she goes for a smear test. It is their responsibility. Remember that, as Jacqui said, 'She's seen the programmes just the same as I have.' If it is sexually transmitted, then she is as likely to have caught it from a former partner as from anything you have passed on to her through him.

Sexual uninterest

Sadly, quite a few women I talked to spoke of general effects on their attitudes to sex, and therefore on their intimate relationships.

'I just went off sex because I had so many internals,' said Heather. 'I don't think we've had a normal sex life since it happened because every time we have intercourse, I bleed,' said Anna. While Linda commented, 'I wouldn't bother if I never had "it" again . . .'

It is sad that this happens. When your feelings about your cervix are altered, by examinations, treatment and the suggestions of a link between disease and your sex life, then your sexuality may well be affected. But it needn't be like this. With more consideration and support from the very beginning, from medical and lay people alike, maybe you can begin to realize that you can separate your cervix from your sexuality – so that one remains intact even if the other is going through a vulnerable time. Some women, in fact, felt that particularly after their treatment, beginning to make love again was part of the healing process.

The men's experience

I spoke to a number of men whose partners had had a positive smear, CIN or cancer. I began by being fairly negative – I had heard so many complaints of men 'not understanding' or 'not listening'. But as the interviews progressed, I realized that what I was hearing was not evidence of male unfeelingness. If anything it was the opposite. What I was hearing was about men who were almost as deeply touched by the experience as their partners were.

Fear or knowledge?

An overriding emotion that many men feel when their partner is ill is fear. And just as we as women are confused and afraid, so can men be. They too can be unsure whether you have cancer or not. Are you going to die? Are they going to lose their partner?

This fear can paralyse. Many women spoke of husbands who could not and would not admit what their condition was: 'I don't think he believed it until we learned I had to have a hysterectomy,' said Diana of her husband. 'He got into his research to a ridiculous extent . . . I realized afterwards that it was because he was worried,' said Heather of her boyfriend.

Even when it becomes clear that your CIN condition is not going to be fatal, your partner may still be frightened. Alain spoke of his real fear that Emma, his wife, might be seriously ill, even though her condition was only CIN 2. 'I burst into tears saying, "Emma might die, Emma might die."'

Remember too that in just the same way as your past experiences have affected your attitude to illness and death, so your partner's past experiences have affected his. Judith's boyfriend had nearly died after a bike accident: 'He thought I was dying, the whole time – and after what he'd been through, he couldn't handle it.' Heather's partner Cedric remembered his grandparents dying of cancer and he was 'very scared.'

Men's fear can come out in different ways from women's fear, because of the different ways we have been brought up. A man may feel uneasy at showing fear, and choose instead to ignore the emotion. He may be angry, he may just deny it is happening, or belittle your illness. 'After all, you haven't got cancer,' Linda's husband said. He may feel that if he gives in to his fear, he will lose face, or be unable to help you with yours.

Just as with women, information can help men to overcome the fear. If a man is informed from the beginning about what is going on and is involved in what is happening, then he will know as much as you will, and will be able to make his own judgements about how serious your condition is. He will be less confused about what CIN means and what it means for you. Many women reported that their partners discussed the hospital leaflets with them, and made great efforts to understand the various stages.

If your condition is serious, and you can talk about this together, then both your fears will find an outlet: 'We did talk seriously about what would happen if I died . . .' said Diana. 'When we heard the news, we talked all night . . . we realized that we'd been very lucky,' said Sue.

Exclusion or involvement?

Men can feel very excluded from what is happening. A man's previous experience of 'women's plumbing problems', as one man sarcastically described his fellow men's approach to things, may have been minimal. And if men don't have the benefit of reading the information, chatting to informed women friends, or facing the medical professionals themselves, then they may well feel excluded and powerless: 'Someone else was helping Heather a lot, and I found this really threatening. I felt inadequate,' said Cedric. 'It was something to do with her body, not with mine,' said Ian.

Many women complained that men didn't get involved – and particularly that they didn't come to hospital appointments as support. If a man, for whatever reason, doesn't feel able to do this – perhaps because he feels he will be in the way – then a vicious circle is created. The more he backs off from involvement, the more he will feel excluded and the less confident he will be.

Some men are able to involve themselves in what is happening. Andrew 'went through all the leaflets with Rachel, discussing what things meant'. Cedric set out to get photocopies of medical articles for his partner to read. Many men were present while their partners had laser treatment, literally holding their hands and giving them support. And the women appreciated this: 'It was really good having him there,' said one woman. 'It made me feel as if we were doing it together.'

Another way in which men can be involved might be to step back from what is happening and leave women to find their own power: 'I was put in a situation where, as Emma's best friend, she wanted me to help her decide whether to have treatment or not . . . but it was such an important decision that I couldn't really be involved in it.' This kind of attitude can seem too objective – but Emma did make her own decision, and was thankful to Alain for letting her make it alone.

Blame or support?

If men are aware of recent press coverage of cervical conditions, then they may feel blamed. If a woman feels that her partner is to blame, then he will certainly feel blamed. 'I know you blame me for it,' said Linda's husband to her – and this reaction was echoed in a number of other accounts.

Whether a man has some cause to feel guilty or not, being blamed may cause him to feel guilty – and angry and resentful. I understand this; we women felt angry and resentful not so long ago when all the blame was being put on us. And if a man cares for his partner, he may feel very threatened by the thought that he has harmed her. As he reacts angrily, she may feel equally threatened, and a cycle of resentment may build up.

So this is one area where men and women can actually ease each other's unhappiness. If the woman doesn't feel bitter, this will allow the man to be more at ease. When I was interviewing Rachel and Andrew, I touched on the question of blame, to be met by genuinely relaxed smiles: 'Well, we talked about that but . . .' It was very obvious that it wasn't an issue for Andrew – because it wasn't an issue for Rachel.

Frustration or acceptance?

Several women reported to me that their husbands were very understanding, until it came to the matter of sex. Men may be angry or frustrated at not being able to make love after their partner's treatment, or at having the spontaneity of sex removed by a change to barrier contraception. There is no reason for either partner to be angry because the other partner will not make love, but as one woman commented wryly, 'My husband's been without for six months, and in normal circumstances he could divorce me for that.'

Particularly if the experience has been bad for you, and you do not feel like making love for a long while, tempers may get frayed. Perhaps for the first time in your relationship, you may need to say 'no' to sex, so that you have time to heal, in every sense of the word. Some women coped with this in their own way. Some were able to make a distinction between love-making with penetration, which they didn't want, and love-making with masturbation, which they felt more at ease with – though as one woman commented to me: 'We didn't get married just to masturbate.'

There are other ways of coping. Viki, at the start of a new relationship, postponed her treatment for two weeks so that she and her new partner could enjoy love-making and stabilize their relationship: 'When the doctor said, "No sex for six weeks," I thought: This is going to wreck it – but I shouldn't have worried as much as I did since my partner was very good and supportive.'

Some women just stated their needs and had them met: 'I went home and said to [my partner], "That's it – from now on you use a condom."' For others of us, who have not been so assertive throughout our relationship, it is difficult to suddenly ask for what we need. And in the area of sex, particularly, we and our men may feel uncomfortable. Many of the men I spoke to had been accepting and supportive, however. Some were happy to wait until their partners felt good about penetrative sex, others spontaneously suggested using barrier contraception: 'He's been very good – we've just got closer and closer, even though we haven't had a normal sex life since it happened,' said Anna.

Independence or vulnerability?

More than one man admitted to needing support – and feeling uneasy about this. For so often, the role men are expected to play in our society is one of supporting the woman. Julie's partner 'seemed to feel he had to be "really strong and manly and I'm here if you want me", rather than dealing with his own feelings about it.'

To complicate matters further, a man may feel that his own need for support should take second place. As Cedric said, 'How can you justify wanting your own support system when your partner hasn't got one? You feel you have to bear it alone.' Many men had found their own way out, by confiding in friends about what was happening. But many are not used to asking for and receiving support, and may not have ready-made support networks.

It is by no means always appropriate for a man to ask his partner for comfort when her condition is serious. Sue's husband's way of coping with her hysterectomy was to tell her constantly, 'Well of course I'm upset about it too,' until one day she lost her temper with him: 'I'm sick and tired of comforting you . . .' She felt better about it, and he learned something from that. But, sometimes if your partner can admit his vulnerability and you can accept it, that alone will enhance your relationship enormously. 'It's just getting better and better,' as one woman said.

Men's experience – what is going on?

The overwhelming impression I got of men both through their own accounts and those of their partners was that they did not mean to hurt women, but did so – unintentionally.

Many men were feeling confused and afraid, threatened and blamed, and reacted by being defensive. They usually shut off their emotions, and retreated into their heads, either because this was the way they were all the time, or because they felt they could not cope. It was not the fact that they didn't realize the seriousness of the situation that made them like this. It was because they *did* appreciate its seriousness and were unable to deal with the implications, while at the same time being 'strong' for their partner. They often admitted to feeling very negative about themselves.

This may not ring true for you. I did hear stories of men behaving in ways which were obviously not motivated by concern: 'I suspect one or two of the girls have had hidings from their husbands over this . . .' was the knowing comment of a woman from a support group in Liverpool. You may, however, like to consider the possibility that where your partner is not able to give you what you want, it is because he is too upset, rather than not upset enough.

So what do we do?

We've looked at things that can go wrong for women in an intimate relationship. We've looked at men's experiences. Often, just being aware of these can help (even if it means you leave this book open at an appropriate page for him/her to read).

Let's end the chapter with a positive statement of what it could be like, based on what men and women I interviewed said they wanted and had often managed to obtain. In what ways can two people in an intimate relationship work together to make the experience a positive one?

Firstly, it could be the chance to really communicate and talk things through. Many couples said that the shock had forced them to do this, and that after the event they had 'kept on talking'. Secondly, you could learn much about each other's needs when under stress: 'I actually needed space to deal with it on my own . . .' said Julie. 'I needed him to come to the hospital with me,' said Rosemary.

You may be able to learn to allow the other person to have their feelings, unimpeded by criticism. Anna comments: 'My partner was great; he never said it's OK, he always said, "it's awful" – and that really helped me because that was what I was feeling too.'

It can be a time of amazingly close physical support; many couples found themselves hugging more than usual, even though their desire to make love was diminished. It can be comforting to know that you don't need to make love in order to be close to each other.

On the practical side, you might learn to use barrier contraception for both your sakes. You might find out you can create intimate relationships that are no less intimate, and no less spontaneous for being risk-free – and that barrier contraception can be a telling sign of what you feel for each other, and how much you care and want to protect each other.

You can get really close by tackling the system together, by going together to examinations, fighting for the treatment you want. You can look back and think: 'We survived that together,' and feel closer because of it.

13

THE PROFESSIONALS

In terms of the treatment I got, I'm satisfied. In terms of
the attitude of the consultant, I'm not. (Frances)

As soon as you enter the system, you come face to face with the
professionals. From the moment you have the smear test, through
the result, the diagnosis and the treatment, they are there. They
guide you, help you and sometimes hinder you. How can you make
the best out of this necessary relationship? How can you turn it into
a positive meeting of equals that gets you back to health as soon as
possible?

Who are the professionals?

Most of the medical professionals we meet fall into three groups.
First are the GPs or local clinic doctors. They are usually the ones
who break the news of a positive smear to us and suggest the next
step. And some of the stories I heard about them were wonderful. Julie's direct question of her doctor: 'Have I got cancer?'
was answered equally directly with a: 'No, you haven't', which
strengthened her for her treatment and cure.

Next, we come into contact with nurses. They are present during
our examination, diagnosis, and treatment. Their role is a little
different. As we shall see, this makes a big difference to the way we
can use them in our attempt to be actively involved in the situation.
Most nurses don't take a directive part in what is happening. They
don't make diagnoses, or suggest treatment. They organize waiting
rooms, support doctors in practical ways, support patients in
emotional ways. In current medical practice, the nurse is there as

your representative in the system, – your advocate to the doctor. 'The nurse was marvellous – she held my hand and kept telling me irrelevant things to take my mind off the treatment,' said one woman.

Finally, we meet the consultant, be it a man or a woman. S/he uses his/her expertise to look, think, pronounce. We know that this person has experience and training. We may feel in awe of them, and we certainly are dependent on them in many ways for the treatment that will give us back our health. Many consultants add to this service by offering the best kind of professional interaction: by being supportive, objective, consultative. 'I really trusted my consultant,' said Rachel. 'He told me the truth.'

What goes right?

At its best, the system works very well. The medical professionals are trained and experienced and they do their job. They take account of your body and your mental state, and work to heal both. There has been a dramatic drop in the death rate for invasive cervical cancer over the last ten years. In the stories I heard, there was example after example of good treatment, of cancer spotted in time, of diagnosis carefully made. Some of the women I interviewed had survived radical invasive cancers.

When the system is really working, your local doctor will talk through with you the need for a smear test and give it to you if necessary. The results, in certain areas of England at any rate, can be received within days. One London GP has even installed a colposcope in her surgery, an example to us all of the system at its best. The diagnosis, treatment and aftercare can run on oiled wheels, as several of my interviewees reported.

There were also examples of superbly good and sensitive meetings with doctors and nurses. One doctor tried to get therapy on the NHS for a patient who hated internal examinations – and supported her in her trying to learn to use a speculum to examine herself. Another 'gave me any amount of time. I could have sat in that room for ever, and he wouldn't have minded,' said Rachel.

What goes wrong?

With the system

The feeling of many women, however, was that the system, the medical health care machine, had in many ways broken down. The resources are not there to make it what it could be. Many of these complaints don't just apply to cervical illnesses or to gynaecological Out-patients wards – but nevertheless, complaints there were.

Firstly of course, there are not enough resources put into screening services. 'Every five years' say the posters – mainly because 'every three years' would put a strain on already tightly stretched resources. Doctors are not paid for testing women under 35, so may fight shy of younger women who come for smears.

Discouraging women from having smears can also occur because there are not the facilities to interpret the results – another consequence of lack of funds. Some areas in the country have three-month waiting lists for smear test results.

Once the results arrive, you wait again. You often have to wait hours in the waiting-room: 'I waited until one o'clock for a ten o'clock appointment,' said one woman. When at last your turn comes, the nurses are often rushing from one place to another and have no time to spend with you. In the consulting room, the same is often true. The doctors have obviously seen many more patients than their energy and attention is up to. They are as exhausted and as stressed as you are. Usually, you don't see the same doctors and nurses every time you attend: 'I went six times and saw someone different on every occasion,' said one woman.

In addition, the system as a whole doesn't seem to take into account how women feel about being examined. Often the procedures for undressing make you feel vulnerable and people other than the consultant will be allowed in to 'take a look' at your condition.

All too often, the waiting list for diagnosis is months long: 'They don't seem to realize the strain it puts on you, not knowing,' said Rosemary. The waiting list for treatment is even longer. And when it is given, in Out-patients, there may not be the facilities to sit down afterwards, to have a hug from your friend or partner, to recover your breath. As an in-patient, you can feel as if you were on a conveyor belt, as overworked nurses shunt you through to make room for tomorrow morning's batch.

Finally, there is no money available for counselling after diagnosis and treatment. Whether that involves cone biopsy, or hysterectomy, laser treatment or a simple diagnosis of the wart virus, there is no professional there to tell you what it means and to listen to your concerns. There is little money available for anything in our system. I'm only too well aware of all the other demands on the resources – but these are the things that we as positive smear women need now.

With the people

In the course of writing this book I found ample evidence of professional and competent conduct, skill and sensitivity, but I was left with the disturbing overall impression that there still seems to be something wrong.

I interviewed nearly thirty women and several of their relatives and received written statements from more, and as I went from interview to interview, it became apparent that the dominant feeling was one of concern. All of these women had been seen, diagnosed, and treated successfully; that was, on the whole, not what they were concerned about. What they were concerned about was not their treatment, but the way in which they had been treated.

I include this preamble because I am not simply using one or two hysterical complaints to make a statement about women's needs. I am, I think, reflecting what many women feel about the way the medical profession reacts to cervical conditions. I am undoubtedly sticking my neck out, but perhaps this will help to change current attitudes.

There were a number of ways in which women thought that they could have been treated better.

The first general complaint was that there was little equal personal contact. Women asked for 'eye contact as I walked in', 'some words aimed at me, not just at the other doctor', 'a response to questions I asked, please.' Others would have appreciated more delicacy: 'Don't walk in on me while I'm undressing,' was one plea.

'I just felt like another pair of spread legs, another piece of research,' commented another woman. These were all appeals for equality, for being treated like another adult with a need for respect. Although this cry is frequently heard in other medical contexts, in this area women perhaps have a more pronounced need.

Some women felt blamed by medical professionals. This is more often due to unfeeling media hype than doctors actually accusing patients face to face. But any number of articles in the medical press contain attacks on women's behaviour. 'Dr X blames permissiveness, promiscuity and the copulation explosion', reads one quote from *The Times*, the speaker an eminent British gynaecologist. It continues, 'I am aware that it might be rather futile advice, but if young women refrained from sex until they were in their twenties . . .' Such statements can only give women the impression that the medical profession is critical of them.

A third worry women had was the powerlessness they had felt when confronted by medical professionals. They had frequently felt excluded from any involvement in their cases and this had been manifested in a number of ways – for example, in the refusal of doctors to give patients information: 'My doctor would not give me my smear result – in the end I went back with my sister and demanded a repeat smear,' said Heather. Few doctors really discussed with patients what was happening, or presented options for treatment. There were, as I have mentioned previously, several cases of patients seeking second opinions to get the treatment they felt was appropriate. And there was also a feeling among women that doctors in general had a vested interest in appearing infallible.

A final thought. Many of the women I spoke to had also had other medical treatment in the past about which they rarely spoke with such concern. It does appear that cervical-related illness is an area which causes women to feel particularly vulnerable, or in which professionals display a particular lack of sensitivity. I am not the first writer to suggest that specializing in gynaecology can be linked with feelings of power in doctors. And perhaps cervical cancer and CIN, where sexuality is so closely linked with disease, is more of a minefield than many other diseases. Dare I suggest that in this area, particularly, doctors may themselves feel ill at ease and unable to communicate with patients, and it is this which causes dissatisfaction on the part of so many patients?

The professionals' point of view

Of course, no argument is ever one-sided. There are reasons to be sympathetic towards the medical profession, and it has to be appreciated that what we as women experience is often not what the professionals *want* us to feel.

Doctors and nurses are only human; they are frequently over-worked and some, particularly the nurses, are drastically under-paid. They work in a very stressful environment. The many professionals I talked to were all extremely committed to eradicating cancer and the stages leading up to it. Most of them were depressed by the unceasing stream of women with cervical conditions that poured through their surgeries and consulting rooms for treatment.

I can understand then the angry frustration of a doctor who thinks he has tracked down a cause and wants people to listen, or the inability of a nurse to keep her patience when there is a three-hour backlog in the waiting-room. I can also understand the unease of a doctor who is not resolved in his or her own mind about sexuality and its place in their own lives, having to treat women whose very condition is a reminder of their sexuality.

Sometimes, particularly with minor CIN conditions, it must be difficult to remember that to the patient, this is a serious matter. It can be hard to understand the emotion of a woman with CIN 1 when the last patient you treated had advanced invasive cancer. Sometimes, too, it must be easy to forget that you are not God when you are making life and death decisions all day and every day.

Medical professionals, like everyone else, are the product of a society that undervalues women. As someone commented: 'If 2,000 men a year died of cancer of the testicles, there would be an outcry.' So perhaps we should understand when women are treated lightly in a medical situation – this is, after all, only a reflection of what happens in the outside world.

I can also imagine many people reading this and thinking that the women I interviewed were biased. After all, they saw the doctor at a time when they were both vulnerable and ill. This is certainly at the heart of the matter. Women are, as one consultant said, 'vulnerable, probably frightened and probably going to be in some discomfort.' But this is, to me, not evidence that women are biased. It is evidence that there needs to be a rethink. Someone needs to get the message through to everyone concerned that it is at this time that women are most in need of care and sensitive handling.

Blame or change?

I have read articles that attack medical attitudes in a far stronger way than I am doing here. This is because I think it is a waste of energy to blame. I would rather use that energy to change. It is my feeling that unless we are all prepared to take responsibility for changing what seems to be happening, then nothing will change. It is hard to expect women to try to change a system when what they are really concerned about is getting themselves better. This is why on many occasions, I suggest taking a supporter or friend with you.

The fact remains that however hard people on the outside try, it is only when people in the system start taking action that attitudes will change. If we as patients can begin to expect to be treated as competent equals, then maybe we will be.

What can we do?

As women

There are lots of practical things we can do to move into a position where we and medical professionals can work together to create health. Many of these have been mentioned in the book where they are relevant, but here is a summary:

The first thing we can do is to make sure that on a physical level we are not vulnerable. As I have mentioned elsewhere, it is possible, and usual now in most hospitals, to be examined without undressing. It is also possible to take a friend in with you during treatment. Some treatments are uncomfortable and some are painful, but as far as you can, take care of your own physical needs, and you will feel more in charge.

The second thing is that we need to become knowledgeable. Knowledge is the doctor's speciality; but if we are able to listen with understanding and ask questions based on that understanding, then we are beginning to be equal. The Facts section of this book contains some of the basics, and throughout the book I suggest questions to ask your doctor.

You can ask to be shown your records, and told about your diagnosis and treatment, if you want to. You do have the choice, though this means you also have the responsibility. You can ask the doctor why s/he is recommending a particular treatment, ask what would happen if other treatments were used, discuss your fears and concerns. You can query his/her decision. Lily's doctor said, 'You have a choice of three treatments . . .'

You can also turn to the nurses for help. They are usually women, and may even have had a positive smear themselves. Current nurses' training teaches that the nurse is an 'advocate' on your behalf. In a fascinating interview with a representative of the Royal College of Nursing, I learnt that 'the patient has personal power, but the nurse has power in the system . . . to plead for the patient.'

A distance will always exist between medical professionals and their patients. Without this protective measure, many doctors would be powerless to help us, because they would be far too involved. But in the case of nurses, the system is organized in such a way that they have the power to support us. Remember, then, that if you feel unsupported, and if you feel powerless, it is not you that is at fault. It means that the system is breaking down.

If all else fails, you can complain about treatment. Your Community Health Council will advise you on your rights and support you in writing to the appropriate body; you will find their number in your phone book.

It is not possible to change the attitudes of all doctors overnight. If you suddenly start questioning and arguing, professionals who have never been questioned in their lives may react negatively. You may be afraid (two or three women were) that if you argue, you will get worse treatment. So don't push yourself beyond your limits.

In taking equal responsibility it must, of course, be borne in mind that once we do, our health is up to us. So if we are going to act as equals, we should take care of ourselves by going for regular smears, taking exercise and eating good food, working with the treatment we decide on and not against it. It's a long-term responsibility and it isn't an easy one.

As professionals

Let me first say that I am aware of the pressures medical professionals are under, and the limitations and lack of resources under which they constantly work.

I am also grateful. Doctors and nurses have saved my life on three occasions, and many of those I have known and met have been wonderful. I also know that a large number of medical professionals who will read this book are innocent of any of the charges I have levelled in this chapter. I'm also aware that a list of things to do won't change anything. Only altering attitudes does that.

But nevertheless, there are some things that medical professionals could fight for, for everyone's sake. They could, for instance, continue to fight within the system for the money and the resources to give more help to positive smear women.

How could this be used? In so many ways. It would be wonderful to whittle down the waiting lists, buy more effective equipment, provide support services to build health before and after treatment. How about a small resource library in each Out-patients waiting-room – so we can learn while we are waiting?

I would also like to make sure that we saw the same doctor and nurses all the time. In one clinic I heard about, there were pictures on the ceiling and music playing while women were being treated. Could we also have professionals spending more time with each patient, to give more information and involve her more fully in the process?

How about a counsellor on hand, after examination, diagnosis, treatment? How about a counsellor on hand to counsel both partners if evidence of the wart virus has been found? Some health authorities are already beginning to introduce this as a regular service.

At the time of going to press, thought is already being given to training for doctors and nurses in what it means for a patient to have a positive smear result. Why not go further and make it standard practice to have patients lecturing them on how it feels to be treated?

There are so many things that could change.

Finally, I shall just ask any medical professionals to do two things: firstly, read this book with an open mind; secondly, the next time you meet a woman with a positive smear condition, and you ask her 'How are you?', stop and wait for the answer, the real answer.

14

SOME PERSONAL STORIES

During the course of writing this book, I interviewed some sixty people and received written accounts or resource material from some thirty more. Of the sixty, over half were women who have had a positive smear, with consequences ranging from no treatment through to radical hysterectomy. Although a large proportion of the ideas, thoughts and examples I have given throughout the book are taken from these women's accounts, I also thought it would be useful to include some more detailed accounts of what happened.

I have chosen these four experiences not because they are dramatic or moving – although they certainly are that. I have chosen them because each, in its own way, is typical of the experiences women related to me. In these four accounts, the main issues – fears, doubts, problems, concerns – of the women I interviewed, are all reflected.

I have edited the original interviews so that they read more or less chronologically and in an ordered way; these edits have been checked and approved by the interviewees. Occasionally, to introduce a topic, I have added an introductory phrase or two; these are always indicated in square brackets. Otherwise these words, thoughts and feelings are the women's own.

Rosemary

I was supposed to have had a smear test in May, and in fact I went in June. I got the letter back very quickly saying come and see us immediately. Then I rushed off to the Family Planning doctor, then to the hospital with the hot little note in my hand, and then of course it just disappeared into the system.

I panicked after a while because I hadn't heard anything about an appointment, and I phoned them up. They said, 'Oh, it's all right. The reason you haven't had an appointment yet is because the consultant doesn't think your case is really urgent – otherwise you'd have been in here by now.' Why didn't they tell me instead of leaving me waiting?

My immediate reaction when I heard the news was sheer terror. I didn't want to talk about it at all. I kept thinking: 'Oh God, I'm going to die. What will happen to the children?' I'm not someone who usually panics, but it was so unexpected.

I had colposcopy and then laser treatment a few months later. It is actually painless, not an unpleasant experience at all, very quick, and the doctors and nurses were very sweet and charming. It was a woman who did the treatment, and she was super, although I have this feeling that if you're older, like I am, they treat you better. But I felt quite sad during it, which I hadn't expected at all. I don't see why it wasn't like giving a pint of blood, even less than that, . . . but it wasn't.

After the treatment, I had intended to go and buy a compost bin. But the friend who came with me, who had had laser treatment before I did, told me to go home instead. I did, and I was glad I did, because I did feel funny, though I don't know why. I wonder whether it was the local anaesthetic? I didn't feel cramps, at least not until later, and I had some bleeding but not much.

[Why do I think I got it?] My doctor said it was the wart virus, and at first I thought: 'Oh that's nothing.' But when my friend explained to me what she'd heard about the wart virus, and what it can do, I was really very shocked. It created real problems for me.

My husband had left about two-and-a-half years ago, and I felt that he was to blame, because he'd had other relationships. I really felt that it was some sort of venereal disease. It's unfair to blame him, because it takes two people to get anything, but I did.

I also felt very worried that I'd had a short sexual affair with somebody who is married, as a real fling when my husband first went off, and I wondered whether I should write and tell this man. The thought of his picking up something from me and giving it to his wife was really quite frightening. I did try to talk to my husband about it a bit, but I probably handled it totally wrongly because I felt quite angry . . . it's quite a difficult thing to talk to somebody about . . .

So when I had to go for treatment, I felt I didn't want any relationships any more. I feel the whole thing is bound up with many areas of your life, not just ones about the cervix.

I think it's changed my attitude to sex in relation to my daughters too. I didn't tell my younger daughter, but I did talk to the older one about it all, though I don't want her to be anxious about it. I hope she avoids going to bed with people early in her life – she's thirteen now.

What I'm left with is a feeling that having a positive smear is a lot like childbirth. It's sexual, it's medical. There are things you can confide in someone who has been through it that you wouldn't confide in someone who hasn't. And it gets to every bit of you . . . you have got to come to terms with the relationship you're having, what's happened to it, your own mortality . . . I think there are a lot of similarities.

Frances

The first time I realized that something was wrong was when I started bleeding after intercourse. It was a good enough excuse for me to go down to the Family Planning Clinic, and they did a smear there, which my GP had never done.

First of all they said I had an erosion on my cervix, which would heal on its own. The bleeding went on for the best part of a year and it got to the stage where I was getting agitated.

Then they sent me to the colposcopy clinic. They did some tests and said there were some pre-cancerous cells and that it would be dealt with by laser treatment at Out-patients.

When I first heard, I did panic. You have great fears of: 'Oh God, my grandmother died of cancer of the womb. Is it hereditary?' Outwardly there wasn't a lot of change really, although I lost a lot of weight. Inwardly though I lost confidence and in some ways I haven't really got it all back. I don't seem to take the initiative; I just seem to draw into myself a lot of the time.

I also wondered what caused it. It seems that they just don't know. I've kept asking them: 'Is it the Pill that's causing it?'

because I've been on the Pill for twelve years and it's probably about time I came off it, what with my being overweight and smoking. But the doctor just says, 'No, you carry on with it.' I haven't found anything that explains particularly well why a positive smear happens. If they told me there was anything I should be doing, then I'd do it, and quite happily. But no one told me to do anything.

The question of how many partners I've had came from the doctor. When I went to the clinic, the doctor said, 'How active a sex life do you have? How many different boyfriends have you had?' as if my sleeping around was the cause of it. I was thinking: 'I've only ever had three boyfriends; is it that bad?'

There was never any question of that from my husband; I know he's had previous partners, he knows I have and I know one of his girlfriends quite well. There's never been any tension on either side about that.

[As for support] I don't suppose I really talked to my husband about it all. I managed to get him to come down to the hospital with me once, but he hates people being ill and can't cope with it. In other ways though he was quite good and understanding.

I haven't met anyone within my circle of friends who has suffered from it, or admits they have. So I doubt that I've told anyone except my sister. When I first had the treatment, she came to the hospital with me and stayed until Ian came home that evening, but other than that I haven't had any support as such.

As for the doctors, in terms of the actual treatment I got, I'm quite satisfied with that. In terms of the attitude of the consultant, I'm not happy about that at all. I did get angry a few times and stood up for myself, and so that was positive.

[Support in terms of information?] I read round after the event but not before. I'm a library assistant – I first searched through our own stock to see if there was anything and there wasn't. There were odd references here and there but they were useless, far too technical.

When the time came to go for the laser treatment, I was frightened. They told me there wouldn't be any side effects, but that's not quite true. I took it easy, but we did go away for a walking trip afterwards, and by the time I got back four days later, I was absolutely exhausted.

My story hasn't really ended. After the first lot of treatment, I was still having the bleeding so they did a D&C. That was eighteen months ago. But it still hasn't been sorted out. I know something is still wrong.

Diana

I had three children and I was pregnant again. It was all planned. I was about thirteen weeks pregnant, and had a smear test, went back two or three weeks later and was told, 'You've got a positive smear, nothing to worry about. You'll be going to a colposcopy clinic, but it's OK.'

That night I came back absolutely fine, thinking there was nothing to worry about. I went to bed, woke up in the middle of the night and thought: 'My God, I'm dying.' It suddenly hit me that having a positive smear must mean that I had cancer.

I rang the hospital the next day and asked whether, if I had cancer, they would call me in immediately. They said of course they would, but when I came off the phone I just cried and cried all day. In the end my husband came home from work because I'd got myself into such a state about it.

When I went for my first examination, the doctor said he thought I would need treatment, but they would wait until I had the baby. There was never a point where I considered not having the baby, because by the time they spotted it, the baby was moving. At each consultation I remember saying to them, 'I've got to have a Caesarian; can't you do a hysterectomy at the same time?' And both the consultant and the registrar kept saying to me, 'You're jumping the gun. It won't come to that.'

My daughter was born in May, and after she was born, I just kept bleeding and was given tablets to stop it. I had my periods and in between 'spotting' practically every day. My fear was that it was an indication that things were more serious than a pre-cancer condition. I went back in September for a colposcopy and biopsy, and then for a cone biopsy. They took away 80 per cent of my cervix. The doctor was wonderful – he went specially to get the results for me and he told me that the results were good and that all the abnormal cells had been removed. I remember thinking: 'Well, this is wonderful. That's it. All over.'

I had a smear a month later which was fine, so by Christmas I thought everything was great. But then I started spotting again, and I went back for another smear and colposcopy.

Two weeks went by, and the doctor hadn't rung me. So I rang him. I asked him the result of my smear, and he said, 'I can't remember.' And then I knew. The next day I got a phone call to say my smear was positive, and would I come in to see another doctor, this time with my husband.

We did that. She explained everything and then she said to me, 'You're thirty. You've had all your children. We think the best thing for you is to have a hysterectomy.' I came away thinking that the main reason to have a hysterectomy was to sterilize me, because of my age and the number of children I had. The doctor obviously found it hard to say that this treatment was necessary because of the abnormal smear. It preyed on my mind that this was not enough reason to have major surgery, so I wrote to the doctor saying I wouldn't have a hysterectomy. Then we saw another doctor who explained to me that in fact there were still abnormal cells in my cervix, in the canal. After that, my husband and I were both convinced that a hysterectomy was the only option, because, if left untreated, the cells would have become invasive cancer.

Then I went into the hospital to have the hysterectomy. I just let go and cried and cried and coped with it that way. The nurses were fantastic, the doctors would come and see me every day and let me ask questions over and over again until I understood. The experience was a positive one in that traumatic period of my life.

It was a hard time. I'm sure most people would feel that. I had been told that everything was clear, and then suddenly I was told that it had come back again. I did lose my trust. But it's all right now.

I did ask why it happened. The media says it is a sexually transmitted disease, and people just hear promiscuity. This was really brought home to me when my mother-in-law rang me one evening saying, 'I was talking to a woman at work who told me that women who get cervical cancer are promiscuous . . .' I was really angry. It can happen to anyone, not necessarily someone promiscuous. We are all at risk once we've had sex.

Also, I was put on the Pill when I was thirteen because of period problems. I keep wondering if that caused it. I didn't have sex until I was twenty-one, so it wasn't early sex . . . I used to smoke as well. But you may never do any of these things, and still get it.

[Support?] The service I had from doctors was good, because I asked for it. I'm confident, fluent and I want to know. We've got to encourage every woman to ask more.

My mother-in-law was great in the end, supportive and terribly worried.

I don't think my husband believed how serious it was; it was only when we heard about my having to have a hysterectomy that he really started to worry. If you ask friends, they would say I wasn't frightened, but with my husband, I'd get really morbid. There was a particular record that my husband bought . . . it will always be very special because it brings back memories of that period of my life, and wondering whether I'd be here the following Christmas.

I think in the end it was quite positive really. I've started doing things, writing leaflets, for the local Health Authority. Many women have said to me that they've found them helpful, and that's good. This all happened about five years ago. I know I'm fine now. I think I'm very lucky.

Evelyn

I wasn't due for a smear. I had one because I went to the Family Planning Clinic because I was taking a new lover.

I had a really good GP who, as soon as he heard, was on the phone to me straight away saying, 'Look my dear, it's important that you go and be seen to immediately. Don't hang about waiting for them. Just go.'

When I went for the examination, I was really impressed by the way the doctor gave time and attention and drew his little diagrams. He explained exactly what was happening and what they would do. It was good.

I had two or three smears, and then I went in for treatment. I had a cylinder biopsy, not a cone, where they take more cells away. I went in on a Tuesday morning and came out on a Friday. I don't really remember much about it. I remember coming out of the anaesthetic and Stanley (my husband) was there . . . then I woke up seemingly four hours later and Helen, my daughter, was there. They'd met in the corridor, so it must have been minutes in between!

Afterwards on the Friday, I went straight from the hospital to do a four-day workshop, and then went straight back to work on the Tuesday.

I don't know what caused it. I thought maybe that it was some kind of continual knocking through intercourse. I certainly haven't drawn any conclusions about numbers of partners. I don't think it could have been that.

At no time did I ever think it was cancer. I knew all the time that it wasn't. I knew from my mother and father that cancer 'is not our thing.' I knew then that none of us would die from that.

It played a very minimal part in my life really. There were a lot of other things going on for me at about the same time, and it just went into the melting pot.

[Support?] Well I did cry, but it's perfectly natural to feel upset. My lover wanted to come and see me in hospital, but we'd just split up, and I wouldn't let him. The doctor was very caring, and the hospital staff were good and at the right level for me, enough information and enough support. I got a lot of attention from people at work, and at the workshop I went to, and I got very close to my daughter when she came to see me in hospital.

It was really no sweat for me, though I think it was a big deal for other people.

15

RESOURCE SECTION

Introduction

This section contains a list of resources which I or other women have found to be useful. They are arranged under subject heading – CIN/Cancer, Smoking etc. Where a resource is relevant to more than one heading, it has been listed more than once. This is to make it easier to use as a reference guide, but it does mean that if you read the text all the way through, it may get a little repetitive! Within each heading, I have listed leaflets, books, people to see, organizations and various other resources such as videos and tapes, so that you can easily find the type of resource you need. To save space, the organizations or contact points have usually been listed by name only and the full address and details are given in the separate address list at the end.

Remember that all details, including prices, may change with time, so it is often useful to check with an organization that their resources are still the same as when this book went to press.

It's noticeable that the majority of the organizations I have listed are in London or the South East. This is sad, but par for the course: nationwide organizations do often base themselves at the centre of communications. I have not been able to track down many provincial support groups for CIN, so if you hear of one, do let me know. The provincial ones for cervical cancer are so numerous that it is probably worth your while approaching a national organization first and asking them for their local group.

A final point. Unfortunately I have not had the opportunity to 'road test' all the resources mentioned here, but all of them have been personally recommended by other women. Even so, mistakes may occur, or you may not receive the good service others did. If you find a resource of organization to be unsatisfactory, do tell them and ask for improvement – and if you like, let me know too. Such information could be incorporated in any future editions of this book. The same applies if you know of a super book, support group or film that isn't mentioned here.

CIN/Cancer

Leaflets

Many hospitals produce their own leaflets, and there are too many to mention here. Ask at your hospital or your Community Health Council for what is available. Addresses of organizations are given at the back of this section.

Understanding Cervical Smears is a sound and helpful 18-page booklet published by BACUP. It explains what a smear is, what further tests can be done and what treatments are used.

Understanding Cancer of the Cervix is a 30-page booklet published by BACUP. It explains what cancer is, how it develops, different treatments and help you can receive. The above two leaflets are provided free to individual callers but organizations are asked to make a donation.

Everyone's Having the Smear Test is a leaflet about what it means to have a test. It is leaflet number 190, available free from the Family Planning Association Information Service.

Cervical Smears: what every woman should know by Anne Szarewski is an informative leaflet about the smear test and colposcopy. It can be obtained from Marie Stopes House free of charge when you attend for diagnosis or treatment.

An Abnormal Smear – what does that mean? An excellent leaflet covering all aspects of having a positive smear and providing information and some advice about what to do. It takes the view that having a positive smear can be a real challenge for women, and highlights some of the emotional issues involved. It costs 20p plus an s.a.e and is available from the Women's Health and Reproductive Rights Information Centre.

Women's Health and Cervical Cancer is an excellent leaflet exploring the issues and giving the facts, from a feminist viewpoint. It is ideal if you want a little more critique with your facts. It also includes a reference section to recent medical texts. The price is 20p plus an s.a.e. from the Women's Health and Reproductive Rights Information Centre.

Cervical cancer – it can be avoided is a leaflet published by the Women's National Cancer Control Campaign. It looks at why we should have smear tests, what they involve and what further examinations may be necessary.

Books

Barker, Graham, *Your Cervical Smear*, Adamson Books, 1987. This is a factual look at smear tests and what happens after them. You may find it useful to fill in more of the medical detail.

Harvey, Judith, Mack, Sue and Wolfson, Julia, *Cervical Cancer and how to Stop Worrying About it*, London, Faber & Faber, 1988 is also factual, but this time based around questions you might ask and concerns you may have.

Both books take a standard viewpoint on the causes of CIN.

People to talk to: one-to-one

There are many organizations offering counselling for all forms of cancer, including cervical cancer. Conversely, there seem to be no tailor-made counselling services for women with CIN, although all the general health organizations and most of the cancer organizations said they would be happy to help. Please note that some organizations and individual counsellors do charge a fee for their services, and you may want to check this ahead of time.

British Association for Counselling can recommend you to a one-to-one counsellor in your area. These counsellors will not usually specialize in medical problems, but can help you talk through your feelings about what is happening; normally counsellors charge fees for their work.

BACUP operates a one-to-one counselling service for cancer patients at their London offices, and are happy to talk about CIN conditions too.

The Bristol Cancer Centre is mainly a residential centre for teaching alternative approaches to cancer, but also provides free information and support on the telephone.

CancerLink has a telephone service which gives you information on cancer and CIN, and on the services they have available.

Cancer Relief provides home nursing and financial support for people with cancer and their families.

Cancer Research Campaign funds research into aspects of all forms of cancer, including cervical cancer. Their research deals with the medical, psychological and social aspects of cancer.

CYANA (Cancer You Are Not Alone) offers a comprehensive service for all types of cancer. This includes one-to-one counselling for sufferers and their families and a 24-hour telephone service.

Dr Jan de Winter Clinic for Cancer Prevention Advice aims to help you minimize the likelihood of contracting cancer, and supports cancer sufferers. It offers free counselling services on a one-to-one basis.

Marie Curie Cancer Care provides nursing in your own home for patients with all forms of cancer. They also run courses for health professionals and cancer research programmes.

Marie Stopes House provides a broad range of gynaecological services for women, including face-to-face counselling.

New Approaches to Cancer offers a referral service for those wanting holistic treatment of all forms of cancer alongside their orthodox treatment. Their service is free, but the counsellor or therapist themselves may charge.

Tak Tent is a Scottish organization of support groups for cancer patients and their families. They also provide a one-to-one counselling service by people trained in counselling those with cancer.

Ulster Cancer Foundation provides information over the phone about all types of cancer.

Women's Health Concern provides a counselling service for women with gynaecological disorders.

The Women's Health and Reproductive Rights Information Centre

runs a phone counselling service for women with CIN and
cervical cancer, and keeps a register of women who have had
treatment and are willing to talk to others.

The Women's National Cancer Control Campaign offers telephone
counselling for all women with cancer, and has a sound knowledge of the problems involved in cervical cancer and CIN
conditions.

People to talk to: support groups

There are a number of support groups for cancer sufferers, though
I could find none specifically for cervical cancer. At the time of
going to press I could find few general ongoing support groups for
women with positive smears. You could try going to an ongoing
cancer support group, but may find that it does not deal only with
cervical conditions. Also, there may be a 'mismatch' between your
situation and the seriousness of the condition of some of the people
in the group.

If you want to start a support group yourself for CIN or cancer
sufferers, CancerLink offers support and training to those starting
groups. *In Our Own Hands*, by Sheila Ernst and Lucy Goodison,
published by The Women's Press, London, 1982 gives some useful
guidelines for running groups.

The Bristol Cancer Centre has 110 support groups countrywide.
Their structure varies, but all are free and all are based round the
philosophy and approach of the Bristol Centre which teaches
self-help and complementary therapies.

CancerLink can put you in touch with support groups in your area,
and provide training and support if you want to set up your own.

Cercan is a support group which was formed after a mix-up over
smears in the Liverpool area resulted in some women being
given a 'negative' result when in fact they had a positive condition. Some later developed more serious cervical conditions.
Cercan is open to all women worried about a positive smear
result. Contact Cercan via Liverpool Community Health
Council, 57/59 Whitechapel, Liverpool LI 6DX, (051-236 1176).

CYANA (Cancer You Are Not Alone) is a centre for sufferers of all types of cancer. The centre is open Monday to Friday inclusive, 10.30–4.00, and support groups take place within those hours.

New Approaches to Cancer is an umbrella for 300 support groups which are mostly free of charge and operate in varying ways, some once a week, some once a month, others on a drop-in basis.

Tak Tent has support groups throughout Scotland and also in England, where you can go and talk through your problems in a supportive atmosphere.

Tapes

The Bristol Cancer Centre offers a wide range of tapes about a complementary health care approach to cancer in general.

Cancer: a positive approach for women is an audio tape about cancer in general written by Linn Branson and recorded by healer Matthew Manning. It is available from the centre, price £5.95 plus 50p postage and packing.

New Approaches to Cancer has a selection of tapes concerned with complementary approaches to all types of cancer.

Videos

Cervical Cancer is a video produced by Leicestershire Health Authority which is relevant to CIN conditions as well as cervical cancer. I have not seen it, but reports are good; however I would suggest viewing it first before using it with a group. It costs £50.00 to buy (£65.00 for U-Matic format) but a 3-day preview can be arranged for £15.00 (£18.00 for U-Matic format). Prices include postage and packing but not VAT. Order from H. & H. Scientific Consultants, PO Box MT27, Leeds LS17 8QP (0532 687189).

Cervical Cancer – The Facts from the Imperial Cancer Research Fund is available from Plymouth Medical Films, Palace Vaults, 33 New Street, Barbican, Plymouth PL12 2NA (0752 267711). It comes with a leaflet and costs £29.95 plus VAT to buy, or £5.50 plus VAT for a seven-day hire. I haven't been able to see or review this film, so you might like to check its relevance to your group before buying it.

New Approaches to Cancer produces a video on new approaches to all forms of cancer.

Test in Time is a video about smear tests prepared by Women's National Cancer Control Campaign. I haven't had a chance to review it.

Down There is a video about the experiences of women after a positive smear; it's funny, hard-hitting and feminist, and ideally should be run with a discussion group afterwards. It's available from Yorkshire Women's Theatre and at time of going to press, the price was £30.00. Cheques should be made payable to Yorkshire Women's Video A/C. See Address list on page 171 for orders.

Other suggestions

Telephone tapes. Healthcall provide a telephone service of recorded health tapes. Ring 01-980 4848 and ask the operator for tape 25 on 'Cervical cancer and cervical smears'; tape 22 for 'Some cancers can be cured' or tape 28 on 'Cancer, what is it?'

Hysterectomy

Leaflets

Many hospitals produce their own leaflets, and there are too many to mention here. Ask at your hospital or your Community Health Council for what is available.

Hysterectomy Support Group produces a leaflet about preparing for and recovering from a hysterectomy, price £1.00.

Hysterectomy and Vaginal Repair is a leaflet written by Sally Haslett and Molly Jennings who have both had hysterectomies. The leaflet covers practical aspects of preparing and recovering from the operation. Send 75p to Beaconsfield Publishers Ltd, Chiltern Hills Road, Beaconsfield, Bucks HP9 1PL. Cheques should be made payable to Beaconsfield Publishers Ltd.

Hysterectomy by Anne Boutwood and Cate Campbell is leaflet number 1 in a series of health booklets from Women's Health Concern and is free from WHC on receipt of an s.a.e.

Books

Druin, Nancy, and Savage, Wendy, *Hysterectomy, what it's all about*, Thames Television, 149 Tottenham Court Road, London WIP 9LL. A large-format leaflet that looks not only at the operation but also at the emotional repercussions.

Henriques, Nikki and Dickson, Anne, *Women on Hysterectomy or How Long Before I Can Hang-Glide*, Wellingborough, Thorsons Publications, 1986. A personal experience book.

People to talk to: one-to-one

The Hysterectomy Support Group was formed to encourage self-help through informal sharing of experience. This can be one-to-one, in telephone counselling or personal meetings. Several of the women I talked to mentioned this group and spoke positively about it. Contact person: Ann Webb.

Women's Health Concern provides counselling for women with gynaecological problems including hysterectomy.

The Women's Health and Reproductive Rights Information Centre has a phone counselling service (see address list for hours of operation). It keeps a register of women who have had a hysterectomy and are willing to talk to others, and will refer to support groups throughout the country.

People to talk to: support groups

The Hysterectomy Support Group. This group has a variety of support groups for women and their partners. It meets in various parts of the country. Contact person: Ann Webb.

Other suggestions

Telephone tapes. Healthcall provide a telephone service of recorded health tapes. Ring 01-980 4848 and ask the operator for tape 148 on 'Hysterectomy'.

Infections and viruses

Leaflets

Herpes Simplex and You is a leaflet compiled by the Herpes Association and contains extracts from many books now out of print; despite this it seems useful. Their information pack containing up-to-date resource material is free on receipt of an s.a.e.

The Herpes Manual (£4.45) and *Stop Herpes Now* (£2.40) are books covering all aspects of having herpes, and are available from the Herpes Association.

All About Genital Warts, Fact Sheet Number 5 is a leaflet giving information on the wart virus and its treatment. It points out the link with cervical conditions and faces up to the problems warts cause in relationships. It is available from the Women's Health and Reproductive Rights Information Centre.

How to Cope with Thrush is a leaflet covering symptoms and treatment of thrush. It is also available from the Women's Health Information Centre.

People to talk to: one-to-one

The Women's Health and Reproductive Rights Information Centre provides a phone counselling service on a wide range of health issues including viruses.

The Herpes Association runs a Helpline for herpes sufferers. They also run a one-to-one counselling service which is free (donation appreciated) and operates by appointment only.

People to talk to: support groups

The Herpes Association runs free support groups for members in various locations, either weekday evenings or Sunday afternoons. Phone them for details of groups in your location.

A support group for women with the wart virus has recently been formed in London. Contact the Women's Health and Reproductive Rights Information Centre for details.

Other suggestions

Telephone tapes. Healthcall provide a telephone service of recorded health tapes. Ring 01-980 4848 and ask the operator for tape 151 on 'Thrush'; 186 on 'Genital warts'; 138 on 'Herpes'.

Contraception

Leaflets

The Family Planning Information Service has a number of short leaflets about all aspects of contraception. They are updated frequently and are all free, although they ask for a contribution to postage. The leaflets include one on contraception (leaflet 020) available in English, Urdu, Punjabi, Bengali, Gujarati and Braille; the basics of birth control (leaflet 041); barrier methods of birth control (leaflet 070); the safe period (leaflet 080); instruction sheet on the condom (leaflet 120); instruction sheet on the cap (leaflet 126); a man's guide to birth control (leaflet 111).

Whose Choice – What Women Have to Say About Contraception is produced by the Oxford Women's Health Action Group (1984). A 42-page booklet giving women's points of view about contraception with information on all methods.

Books

There are a number of books on contraception, and it is difficult to recommend just one. The following have been mentioned to me as being particularly helpful by women I have spoken to.

Shapiro, Rose, *Contraception: a practical and political guide*, London, Virago, 1987. A full and aware book; it may be a little heavy going if all you want to know are the basics.

Boston Women's Health Book Collective, *The New Our Bodies Ourselves*, New York, Simon & Schuster, 1987. Covers all forms of contraception in detail and gives a feminist perspective.

People to talk to: one-to-one

Your local GP or Family Planning Clinic will usually be able to give you advice and support on methods of contraception, and on moving from one method to another.

The Women's Health and Reproductive Rights Information Centre offer a phone counselling service on a wide range of health issues including contraception. They also provide an information pack on contraception, for use with support groups and lectures.

Marie Stopes House provides a broad range of services for women including contraception and counselling. Note that Marie Stopes House is a private clinic and you will have to pay for your treatment.

Other suggestions

Telephone tapes . Healthcall provide a telephone service of recorded health tapes. Ring 01-980 4848 and ask the operator for tape 64 on 'Contraception for Men', 68 on 'Contraception for Women', and 66 on 'The Pill'.

General health

Leaflets

The Women's Health and Reproductive Rights Information Centre provides a variety of leaflets about all aspects of women's health, including food, alcohol, housing and stress. For a full list write to them directly; each leaflet costs 20p plus postage and packing.

Books

Girling, Richard (ed.), *Sunday Times Lifeplan*, London, Collins, 1987. This is the book of the series of excellent articles featured in the Sunday Times. It takes an interactive approach to health, encouraging you to look at what you are doing now, and how you could improve your lifestyle.

Boston Women's Health Book Collective, *The New Our Bodies Ourselves*, New York, Simon & Schuster, 1987. The new version of the old feminist favourite is even better than the original, with a comprehensive listing of all general health issues, and sections on issues particularly relevant to positive smears, cervical cancer, viruses and contraception.

People to talk to: one-to-one

The Women's Health and Reproductive Rights Information Centre offers a phone counselling service (times given in address list) on a wide range of health issues. The phones are always answered by women, who understand women's problems and will do their best to advise and refer where necessary.

Other suggestions

Telephone tapes . Healthcall provide a telephone service of recorded health tapes. Ring 01-980 4848 and ask the operator for tape 119 on 'Fibre'.

Smoking

Leaflets

ASH have a number of leaflets about stopping smoking, including 'Smoking and Reproduction' and 'The health consequences of smoking for women'. They are 10p each from ASH.

Women and Smoking, a general leaflet about women's health, price 20p plus an s.a.e. from the Women's Health and Reproductive Rights Information Centre.

Books

Women and Smoking – A Handbook for Action is a resource guide from ASH and the Health Education Authority. Price £2.00 from ASH.

Jacobson, Dr Bobbie, *Beating the Ladykillers*, London, Pluto, 1986 includes helpful ideas on how women can give up smoking.

People to talk to: one-to-one

The Women's Health Information Centre offers a phone counselling service at the times mentioned on a wide range of health issues including smoking.

People to talk to: support groups

ASH has support groups throughout the country for those giving up smoking.

Other suggestions

Give Up Pack from ASH includes information on the hazards of smoking and handy tips on how to give up for good. Details from ASH.

Telephone tapes. Healthcall provide a telephone service of recorded health tapes. Ring 01-980 4848 and ask the operator for tape 133 on 'Smoking and how to give up'.

Complementary medicine

Leaflets

The Bristol Cancer Centre produce a number of leaflets on complementary approaches to cancer care, including some on their special diet, relaxation and meditation, and Bach Flower Remedies. A full list of leaflets and their prices can be obtained by contacting BCC direct.

New Approaches to Cancer. A leaflet on alternative and holistic approaches to cancer is available if you send them an s.a.e.

Alternative Medicine: promoting Good Health. A leaflet about the alternatives to orthodox approaches. It is available from the Women's Health and Reproductive Rights Information Centre.

Books

There are many books on complementary medicine. The following organizations have book lists:

The Yearbook of the Institute of Complementary Medicine includes nationwide listings of services in each of the main complementary disciplines. It also lists counselling services and patient support groups. It costs £5.95 or £6.30 postage and packing, and is available from the ICM.

New Approaches to Cancer and *The Bristol Cancer Centre* both offer a selection of books on holistic approaches to cancer. They will send you a list on receipt of an s.a.e.

Boston Women's Health Book Collective, *The New Our Bodies Ourselves*, New York, Simon & Schuster, 1987. Has a comprehensive listing of all general health issues, often with an alternative slant.

People to talk to: one-to-one

Awakenings provides a counselling and support service, and will also refer you to local complementary medicine practitioners. It has links with the healer Matthew Manning and special expertise in dealing with cancer.

The Bristol Cancer Centre is mainly a residential centre for teaching alternative approaches to cancer. It also provides free information and support on the telephone.

The Institute of Complementary Medicine has lists of counsellors trained in complementary approaches, and you can obtain details by ringing them. They also have 72 volunteer-manned Public Information Points which provide local information about complementary medicine.

New Approaches to Cancer offers a referral service for those wanting holistic treatment of all forms of cancer alongside their orthodox treatment and will refer you to a local counsellor if you wish. Their service is free, but the counsellor or therapist may charge – you can check beforehand or ask them to refer you to a free service.

The Women's Health and Reproductive Rights Information Centre offers a phone counselling service on a wide range of health issues and will advise you on complementary medicine if they can.

People to talk to: support groups

The Bristol Cancer Centre has 110 support groups nationwide. Their structure varies, but all are free and all are based round the philosophy and approach of the Bristol Centre which teaches self-help and complementary therapies.

The Institute of Complementary Medicine has lists of patient support groups throughout the country. Ring them for details.

New Approaches to Cancer refers those with all forms of cancer who wish to use holistic approaches alongside orthodox medical treatment. They are an umbrella for 300 support groups which are mostly free of charge and operate in various ways, some once a week, some once a month, others on a drop-in basis. Contact NAC for details of your local group.

Tapes

The Bristol Cancer Centre offers a wide range of tapes about a complementary health care approach to cancer in general.

Cancer: a positive approach for women is an audio tape written by Linn Branson and recorded by healer Matthew Manning. It is available from the centre, price £5.95 plus 50p postage and packing.

New Approaches to Cancer offers a selection of tapes concerned with complementary approaches to all types of cancer.

Videos

New Approaches to Cancer has a video on new approaches to all forms of cancer. Available on sale or for hire.

Other suggestions

Telephone tapes. Healthcall provide a telephone service of recorded health tapes. Ring 01-980 4848 and ask the operator for tape 160 on 'Acupuncture', 162 on 'Homoeopathy'.

Organizations

Cancer Research Campaign funds research into aspects of all forms of cancer, including cervical cancer.

Community Health Councils. Your local one will usually be able to put you in touch with local support groups, health information services, and pressure groups. If you have problems with medical practitioners, they will support you to obtain your rights. Find them in your phone book or Yellow Pages.

WACC! (Women Against Cervical Cancer) is a pressure and fundraising group which aims to improve NHS facilities for diagnosing and treating cancer. It wants to start fund-raising groups nationwide for cervical cancer diagnosis and treatment in the NHS.

Address list

Ash, 5–11 Mortimer Street, London WIN 7RH (01-637 9843; Mon.–Fri. 9.30–5.30).

Association for Neuro-Linguistic Programming, c/o 100b Carysfort Road, London N16.

Awakenings, 18c Marylands Road, Maida Vale, London W9 2DV (01-289 8305; Mon.–Fri. 1.00–6.00, or ansaphone).

British Association for Counselling, 37a Sheep Street, Rugby, Warwickshire CV21 3BX (0788-78328/9; office hours, then ansaphone).

BACUP, British Association of Cancer United Patients and their Families and Friends, 121/123 Charterhouse Street, London EC1M 6AA (01-608 1661; 5 lines).

The Bristol Cancer Help Centre, Grove House, Cornwallis Grove, Clifton, Bristol BS8 4PG (0272-743216).

CancerLink, 46 Pentonville Road, London N1 9HF (01-833 2451; Mon.–Fri. 9.30–5.30, ansaphone at other times).

Cancer Relief, 15–19 Britten Street, London SW3 3TZ (01-351 7811).

Cancer Research Campaign, 2 Carlton House Terrace, London SW1Y 5AR (01-930 8972).

Co-Counselling International, c/o Cris Nikolov, 79a Ferme Park Road, London N8 9SA.

Community Health Councils. Find them in your phone book or Yellow Pages.

CYANA (Cancer You Are Not Alone), 31 Church Road, London E12 6AD (01-533 5366; office hours and 01-472 8861; after hours).

The Family Planning Association, 27/35 Mortimer Street, London WIN 7RJ (01-636 7866; weekdays 9.00–5.00; Fri. 9.00–4.30, ansaphone after this).

The Herpes Association, 41 North Road, London N7 9DP (01-609 9061; 24 hours).

The Hysterectomy Support Group, 11 Henryson Road, Brockley, London SE4 1HL (01-690 5987).

The Imperial Cancer Research Fund, 26 Victoria Road, Surbiton, Surrey KT6 4JZ (01-390 6659).

ICM, (The Institute for Complementary Medicine), 21 Portland Place, London WIN 3AF (01-636 8543; office hours, seven days a week).

The Dr Jan de Winter Clinic for Cancer Prevention Advice, 6 New Road, Brighton, Sussex BNI 1UF (0273-727213; 10.00–4.00 and 0323-870500; after hours).

Marie Curie Cancer Care, 28 Belgrave Square, London SWIX 8QG (01-235 3325; weekdays 8.30–5.30).

Marie Stopes House, 108 Whitfield Street, London WIP 6BE (01-388 0662; office hours).

Matthew Manning Centre, 39 Abbeygate Street, Bury St Edmunds, Suffolk IP33 1LW (0284-69502/752364; Mon.–Fri. 9.00–5.30).

New Approaches to Cancer, c/o The Seekers Trust, Addington Park, Maidstone, Kent ME19 5BL (0732-848336; Mon.–Fri. 9.00–5.00, then ansaphone).

Tak Tent, contact through Beatson Oncology Centre, Western Infirmary, Glasgow GI1 6NT (041-339 8822).

Ulster Cancer Foundation, 40–42 Eglantine Avenue, Belfast BT9 6DX (0232-663281).

WACC! (Women Against Cervical Cancer), 4 Grosvenor Cottages, Eaton Terrace, London SWI 8NA.

Women's Health Concern, Ground Floor, 17 Earls Terrace, London W8 6LP (01-602 6669).

Women's Health and Reproductive Rights Information Centre, 52 Featherstone Street, London ECI1 8RT (01-251 6580: Mon., Tues., Thurs., Fri. 12.00–4.00; Wed. 2.00–6.00).

Women's National Cancer Control Campaign, 1 South Audley Street, London WI1 5DQ (01-499 7532; weekdays 9.00–5.00, then ansaphone).

Yorkshire Women's Theatre, Yorkshire Women's Video, 86 Mexborough Grove, Leeds LS7 3EA (0532-490691). To purchase their video, cheques should be sent to: Julie Courtney, 50 Karnak Road, Leeds 6SE 5JS.

16

QUESTIONS TO ASK

_____

This is a summary of the questions you could ask your doctor or consultant at various stages of your diagnosis and treatment. They are all given at appropriate places in the book, but I have gathered them together here for easy reference.

Questions to ask your GP or Family Planning Clinic if you see them after your positive smear:

> What is my smear test result?
> What severity of dyskaryosis have I got?
> Is there any other evidence to indicate what my condition is?
> Is there any sign of infection? A virus?
> Do I need to see a consultant? When? Where?
> How will the appointment be made?
> Do I need to come back to you for a repeat smear? When?
> Should I make the appointment now?

Questions to ask the consultant when you go for further examination:

> What is your name? What sort of doctor are you? What job do you do in the hospital?
> What is the nurse's name? Will she stay in the room with me?
> What has my GP said to you in his letter?
> Are you going to do another smear? A colposcopy? A punch biopsy?
> Will there be anyone else in the room while I'm being examined?

Questions to ask your consultant after a colposcopy/punch biopsy, or at diagnosis stage:

What exactly did you find during the colposcopy?

What was my repeat smear result?

What did the punch/cone biopsy show?

What grade of CIN do I have?

How far has it spread?

Can you tell me now whether my condition is cancerous or pre-cancerous?

Questions to ask your doctor or consultant about inflammations, infections or viruses:

Did you notice any inflammation in my cervix; do you know what might be causing this?

Was there any vaginal discharge? Can you suggest what might be causing this?

Did you find any evidence of a viral infection, particularly the wart virus?

Questions to ask a consultant concerning the treatment s/he suggests:

What treatment do you think would be best for me?

Why are you choosing this sort of treatment?

What will be the after effects of this treatment (on my ability to have children, make love, etc)?

Will my treatment mean my changing methods of contraception (will I have to have my IUCD removed)?

What would be the position if I wanted to have . . . (any other form of treatment than the one the doctor has mentioned)?

Why would you not recommend this?

I am concerned about these things; could I talk them through with you?

When would you treat me?

Will I be an out-patient? (If so, when, for how long?)

Will I be an in-patient? (If so, when, for how long?)

LAST WORDS

————————

Towards the end of each interview I asked all the women this question: 'What do you want to say to the people who read this book?' This is what they replied:

It's a problem that concerns women; it's not caused by women. (Diana)

Keep going, everything is going to be OK. Don't feel dirty, or guilty. Don't panic. Fight for what's best for you. (Heather)

The operation is only a day of pain; it can be got rid of. (Rachel)

Cheer up. It's not that bad. You're getting through it. (Janet)

Take notice. Women should get together. (Emma)

In the last resort, I wasn't just a cervix. I didn't have to do what I was told. (Jane)

Loads of people have it, loads of people have to go through it . . . no problem. (Jo)

Just keep asking the questions . . . just keep pushing. (Rosemary)

Make sure you get looked after. (Evelyn)

Look! It happened to me and I'm OK! (Jane B.)

NOTES

1. Richardson, A. C. and Lyon, J. B., 'The Effect of Condom Use on Squamous Cell Cervical Intraepithelial Neoplasia', *American Journal of Obstetrics and Gynecology*, vol. 140, No. 8 (1981), 909ff.

2. Richardson, A. C. and Lyon, J. B., *op. cit.*

3. Dr Peter Skrabenek, as reported in the *Irish Medical Times*, 14 March 1986.

4. Robinson, Jean, 'Cancer of the Cervix: Occupational Risks of Husbands and Wives and Possible Preventative Strategies', in *Pre-Clinical Neoplasia of the Cervix, Proceedings of the Ninth Study Group of the Royal College of Obstetricians and Gynaecologists*, Jordan, J. A., Sharp, F. and Singer, A. (eds.), (Royal College of Obstetricians and Gynaecologists: London 1982), 11–27.

5. Harris, R. W. C. *et al.*, 'Characteristics of Women with Dysplasia or Carcinoma in Situ of the Cervix', *British Journal of Cancer*, vol. 42 (1980), 359.

6. Gagnon, F., 'Contribution to the Study of the Etiology and Prevention of Cancer of the Cervix and of the Uterus', *American Journal of Obstetrics and Gynecology*, vol. 60 (1950), 516.

7. These theories are based on a number of studies carried out over the past fifteen years, as reported in most basic gynaecological textbooks, e.g. Boon, Matilde E. and Tabbers–Boumeester, Mette–Lise, *Gynaecological Cytology* (London: Macmillan, 1980).

8. See correspondence in *The Lancet*, 25 April 1987, McCance, D. J., 'Human Papilloma Virus and Cervical Cancer'.

9. Meanwell, C. A. *et al.*, 'HPV-16 DNA in Normal and Malignant Cervical Epithelium: Implications for the Aetiology and Behaviour of Cervical Neoplasia', *The Lancet*, 28 March 1987. See also the editorial of the same issue: '. . . the case against the papilloma viruses is far from proven . . .'

10. Wickenden, C., *et al.*, 'Prevalence of HPV, DNA and viral copy

numbers in cervical scrapes from women with normal and abnormal cervices', *Journal of Pathology*, vol. 153 (1987), 127–35.

11. Murdoch, J. B., Cordiner, J. W. and MacNab, J. C. M., 'Relevance of HPV-16 to laser therapy for cervical lesions', *The Lancet*, 20 June 1987.

INDEX

sex and 28

questions 172–3
  on diagnosis 30–31, 173
  doctor's 21–2
  at examination 21, 172
  on smear test results 13, 172
  on treatment 50, 173

radical treatment 60–68
radio, networks and 123–4
radiotherapy 49, 66–7
rape, past 105, 108
reactions
  emotional: to CIN diagnosis 33;
    delayed 9; to examination 28;
    partner's 130–35; to positive
    smear 1, 2, 8–9, 13–14, 15–16,
    126–30; to treatment 54, 55–6,
    60
  physical: to examination 27–8; to
    treatment 54–5, 59–60
recalls 77
recovery
  from examination 27–8
  from treatment 54, 57, 59–60:
    radical 65, 67, 68
referral, specialist 12
reflexology 44
re-infection 75
relationships, intimate 125–36
  traumatic 105
  see also partner
relatives, fear of 61
relaxation 15–16, 39, 71
  and complementary medicine 44
  before/after treatment 52, 54, 57
remission, spontaneous 32
  with condom use 40
  of viruses 42
repeat smear 12, 14
  and condom use 40
reproductive system 81–2
Rescue Remedy 51
resources 80, 155–71
  lack of medical 98, 139, 140, 145
  for support groups 122
responses see reactions
results
  examination 29

forms 92
  obtaining test 11–13
  possibility of wrong 10
  repeat smear 14
rights, patient 35–6, 144
risk factors 95–106
rogue sperm 129

safe period 72, 74, 164
sanitary towels, need for
  at examination 21, 27
  at treatment 51, 54, 55, 57
scans, cancer 62–3
screening 76–8
  camera 93
  lack of resources in 139
second opinions 35
'secondaries' 87
self-cure, failure of 109
self-esteem 107–15
self-help 169, 170
  for wart virus 43
sex
  abstinence from 76
  age and 101, 102
  biology of 82
  bleeding after 149
  change in attitude to 129–30,
    149
  after CIN treatment 55, 59
  doctors' views of 141
  embarrassment about 119
  after examination 28
  hygiene and 72
  after hysterectomy 65
  pain during 30
  partners see partners
  Pill and 100
  and responsibility 128
  self-blame and 110–11
sexual behaviour
  and cancer/CIN 3, 74–5, 100–2
  doctors' questions on 22
  male 128–9
sexual relationships 125–36
sexual triggers, possible 102–4
sexually transmitted disease
    (STD) 42, 99, 103, 128
  embarrassment about 119
shock 8, 38, 51

FOR THE BEST IN PAPERBACKS, LOOK FOR THE

In every corner of the world, on every subject under the sun, Penguin represents quality and variety – the very best in publishing today.

For complete information about books available from Penguin – including Pelicans, Puffins, Peregrines and Penguin Classics – and how to order them, write to us at the appropriate address below. Please note that for copyright reasons the selection of books varies from country to country.

In the United Kingdom: Please write to *Dept E.P., Penguin Books Ltd, Harmondsworth, Middlesex, UB7 0DA*

In the United States: Please write to *Dept BA, Penguin, 299 Murray Hill Parkway, East Rutherford, New Jersey 07073*

In Canada: Please write to *Penguin Books Canada Ltd, 2801 John Street, Markham, Ontario L3R 1B4*

In Australia: Please write to the *Marketing Department, Penguin Books Australia Ltd, P.O. Box 257, Ringwood, Victoria 3134*

In New Zealand: Please write to the *Marketing Department, Penguin Books (NZ) Ltd, Private Bag, Takapuna, Auckland 9*

In India: Please write to *Penguin Overseas Ltd, 706 Eros Apartments, 56 Nehru Place, New Delhi, 110019*

In Holland: Please write to *Penguin Books Nederland B.V., Postbus 195, NL–1380AD Weesp, Netherlands*

In Germany: Please write to *Penguin Books Ltd, Friedrichstrasse 10–12, D–6000 Frankfurt Main 1, Federal Republic of Germany*

In Spain: Please write to *Longman Penguin España, Calle San Nicolas 15, E–28013 Madrid, Spain*

In France: Please write to *Penguin Books Ltd, 39 Rue de Montmorency, F-75003, Paris, France*

In Japan: Please write to *Longman Penguin Japan Co Ltd, Yamaguchi Building, 2–12–9 Kanda Jimbocho, Chiyoda-Ku, Tokyo 101, Japan*

PENGUIN HEALTH

Audrey Eyton's F-Plus   Audrey Eyton

'Your short cut to the most sensational diet of the century' – *Daily Express*

Baby and Child   Penelope Leach

A beautifully illustrated and comprehensive handbook on the first five years of life. 'It stands head and shoulders above anything else available at the moment' – Mary Kenny in the *Spectator*

Woman's Experience of Sex   Sheila Kitzinger

Fully illustrated with photographs and line drawings, this book explores the riches of women's sexuality at every stage of life. 'A book which any mother could confidently pass on to her daughter – and her partner too' – *Sunday Times*

Food Additives   Erik Millstone

Eat, drink and be worried? Erik Millstone's hard-hitting book contains powerful evidence about the massive risks being taken with the health of the consumer. It takes the lid off the food we have and the food industry.

Living with Allergies   Dr John McKenzie

At least 20% of the population suffer from an allergic disorder at some point in their lives and this invaluable book provides accurate and up-to-date information about the condition, where to go for help, diagnosis and cure – and what we can do to help ourselves.

Living with Stress   Cary L. Cooper, Rachel D. Cooper and Lynn H. Eaker

Stress leads to more stress, and the authors of this helpful book show why low levels of stress are desirable and how best we can achieve them in today's world. Looking at those most vulnerable, they demonstrate ways of breaking the vicious circle that can ruin lives.

Medicines: A Guide for Everybody   Peter Parish

This sixth edition of a comprehensive survey of all the medicines available over the counter or on prescription offers clear guidance for the ordinary reader as well as invaluable information for those involved in health care.

Pregnancy and Childbirth   Sheila Kitzinger

A complete and up-to-date guide to physical and emotional preparation for pregnancy – a must for all prospective parents.

The Penguin Encyclopaedia of Nutrition   John Yudkin

This book cuts through all the myths about food and diets to present the real facts clearly and simply. 'Everyone should buy one' – *Nutrition News and Notes*

The Parents' A to Z   Penelope Leach

For anyone with a child of 6 months, 6 years or 16 years, this guide to all the little problems involved in their health, growth and happiness will prove reassuring and helpful.

Jane Fonda's Workout Book

Help yourself to better looks, superb fitness and a whole new approach to health and beauty with this world-famous and fully illustrated programme of diet and exercise advice.

Alternative Medicine   Andrew Stanway

Dr Stanway provides an objective and practical guide to thirty-two alternative forms of therapy – from Acupuncture and the Alexander Technique to Macrobiotics and Yoga.

PENGUIN HEALTH

The Prime of Your Life   Dr Miriam Stoppard

The first comprehensive, fully illustrated guide to healthy living for people aged fifty and beyond, by top medical writer and media personality, Dr Miriam Stoppard.

A Good Start   Louise Graham

Factual and practical, full of tips on providing a healthy and balanced diet for young children, *A Good Start* is essential reading for all parents.

How to Get Off Drugs   Ira Mothner and Alan Weitz

This book is a vital contribution towards combating drug addiction in Britain in the eighties. For drug abusers, their families and their friends.

Naturebirth   Danaë Brook

A pioneering work which includes suggestions on diet and health, exercises and many tips on the 'natural' way to prepare for giving birth in a joyful relaxed way.

Pregnancy   Dr Jonathan Scher and Carol Dix

Containing the most up-to-date information on pregnancy – the effects of stress, sexual intercourse, drugs, diet, late maternity and genetic disorders – this book is an invaluable and reassuring guide for prospective parents.

Care of the Dying   Richard Lamerton

It is never true that 'nothing more can be done' for the dying. This book shows us how to face death without pain, with humanity, with dignity and in peace.

PENGUIN HEALTH

Acupuncture for Everyone   Dr Ruth Lever

An examination of one of the world's oldest known therapies used by the Chinese for over two thousand years.

Aromatherapy for Everyone   Robert Tisserand

The use of aromatic oils in massage can relieve many ailments and alleviate stress and related symptoms.

Chiropractic for Everyone   Anthea Courtenay

Back pain is both extremely common and notoriously difficult to treat. Chiropractic offers a holistic solution to many of the causes through manipulation of the spine.

Herbal Medicine for Everyone   Michael McIntyre

An account of the way in which the modern herbalist works and a discussion of the wide-ranging uses of herbal medicine.

Homoeopathy for Everyone   Drs Sheila and Robin Gibson

The authors discuss the ways in which this system of administering drugs – by exciting similar symptoms in the patient – can help a range of disorders from allergies to rheumatism.

Hypnotherapy for Everyone   Dr Ruth Lever

This book demonstrates that hypnotherapy is a real alternative to conventional healing methods in many ailments.

Osteopathy for Everyone   Paul Masters

By helping to restore structural integrity and function, the osteopath gives the whole body an opportunity to achieve health and harmony and eliminate ailments from migraines to stomach troubles.

Spiritual and Lay Healing   Philippa Pullar

An invaluable new survey of the history of healing that sets out to separate the myths from the realities.

FOR THE BEST IN PAPERBACKS, LOOK FOR THE 🐧

A CHOICE OF PENGUINS AND PELICANS

Metamagical Themas Douglas R. Hofstadter

A new mind-bending bestseller by the author of *Gödel, Escher, Bach*.

The Body Anthony Smith

A completely updated edition of the well-known book by the author of *The Mind*. The clear and comprehensive text deals with everything from sex to the skeleton, sleep to the senses.

How to Lie with Statistics Darrell Huff

A classic introduction to the ways statistics can be used to prove *anything*, the book is both informative and 'wildly funny' – *Evening News*

The Penguin Dictionary of Computers Anthony Chandor and others

An invaluable glossary of over 300 words, from 'aberration' to 'zoom' by way of 'crippled lead-frog tests' and 'output bus drivers'.

The Cosmic Code Heinz R. Pagels

Tracing the historical development of quantum physics, the author describes the baffling and seemingly lawless world of leptons, hadrons, gluons and quarks and provides a lucid and exciting guide for the layman to the world of infinitesimal particles.

The Blind Watchmaker Richard Dawkins

'Richard Dawkins has updated evolution' – *The Times* 'An enchantingly witty and persuasive neo-Darwinist attack on the anti-evolutionists, pleasurably intelligible to the scientifically illiterate' – Hermione Lee in Books of the Year, *Observer*

FOR THE BEST IN PAPERBACKS, LOOK FOR THE 🐧

A CHOICE OF PENGUINS AND PELICANS

Genetic Engineering for Almost Everybody   William Bains

Now that the 'genetic engineering revolution' has most certainly arrived, we all need to understand the ethical and practical implications of genetic engineering. Written in accessible language, they are set out in this major new book.

Brighter than a Thousand Suns   Robert Jungk

'By far the most interesting historical work on the atomic bomb I know of' – C. P. Snow

Turing's Man   J. David Bolter

We live today in a computer age, which has meant some startling changes in the ways we understand freedom, creativity and language. This major book looks at the implications.

Einstein's Universe   Nigel Calder

'A valuable contribution to the de-mystification of relativity' – *Nature*

The Creative Computer   Donald R. Michie and Rory Johnston

Computers *can* create the new knowledge we need to solve some of our most pressing human problems; this path-breaking book shows how.

Only One Earth   Barbara Ward and Rene Dubos

An extraordinary document which explains with eloquence and passion how we should go about 'the care and maintenance of a small planet'.

FOR THE BEST IN PAPERBACKS, LOOK FOR THE 🐧

A CHOICE OF PENGUINS AND PELICANS

The Informed Heart   Bruno Bettelheim

Bettelheim draws on his experience in concentration camps to illuminate the dangers inherent in all mass societies in this profound and moving masterpiece.

God and the New Physics   Paul Davies

Can science, now come of age, offer a surer path to God than religion? This 'very interesting' (*New Scientist*) book suggests it can.

Modernism   Malcolm Bradbury and James McFarlane (eds.)

A brilliant collection of essays dealing with all aspects of literature and culture for the period 1890–1930 – from Apollinaire and Brecht to Yeats and Zola.

Rise to Globalism   Stephen E. Ambrose

A clear, up-to-date and well-researched history of American foreign policy since 1938, Volume 8 of the Pelican History of the United States.

The Waning of the Middle Ages   Johan Huizinga

A magnificent study of life, thought and art in 14th and 15th century France and the Netherlands, long established as a classic.

The Penguin Dictionary of Psychology   Arthur S. Reber

Over 17,000 terms from psychology, psychiatry and related fields are given clear, concise and modern definitions.